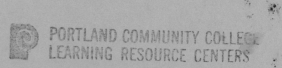

Claire's Classic American Vegetarian Cooking

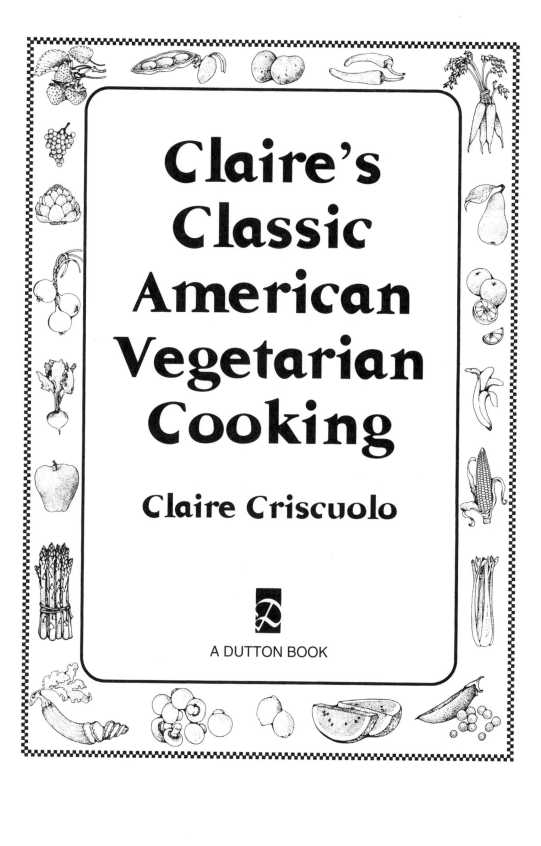

Claire's Classic American Vegetarian Cooking

Claire Criscuolo

A DUTTON BOOK

DUTTON
Published by the Penguin Group
Penguin Books USA Inc., 375 Hudson Street,
New York, New York, 10014, U.S.A.
Penguin Books Ltd, 27 Wrights Lane,
London W8 5TZ, England
Penguin Books Australia Ltd, Ringwood,
Victoria, Australia
Penguin Books Canada Ltd, 10 Alcorn Avenue,
Toronto, Ontario, Canada M4V 3B2
Penguin Books (N.Z.) Ltd, 182–190 Wairau Road,
Auckland 10, New Zealand

Penguin Books Ltd, Registered Offices:
Harmondsworth, Middlesex, England

First published by Dutton, an imprint of Dutton Signet, a division of Penguin Books USA Inc.
Distributed in Canada by McClelland & Stewart Inc.

First Printing, April, 1997
10 9 8 7 6 5 4 3 2 1

 REGISTERED TRADEMARK—MARCA REGISTRADA

LIBRARY OF CONGRESS CATALOGING-IN-PUBLICATION DATA:

Criscuolo, Claire.
   [Classic American vegetarian cooking]
   Claire's classic American vegetarian cooking / Claire Criscuolo.
      p.   cm.
   ISBN 0-525-94179-7 (alk. paper)
   1. Vegetarian cookery. 2. Cookery, American. 3. Claire's Corner Copia (Restaurant)
I. Title.
TX837.C772   1997
641.5 '636—dc20   96-34726
                                                                CIP

Printed in the United States of America
Set in Sabon
Designed by Leonard Telesca

This book is lovingly dedicated to
Lisa, Branden, Carley, and Carolyn LaPia,
four of the greatest joys of my life.

Acknowledgments

I owe a huge debt of gratitude to so many wonderful people who helped make this book possible. I should first thank my mother for raising my brothers and me in a loving home where delicious food was lavished on us. She instilled in us a love and respect for good, wholesome food, and taught us to respect and recognize quality.

It seems like only yesterday that I was writing my first book, *Claire's Corner Copia Cookbook*, but more than two years have passed. **Claire's Corner Copia**, my beloved vegetarian restaurant, celebrated its twentieth anniversary (where did the time go?) on September 17, 1995. Donald Jackson, Javier Lopez, Rose Albin, Mike Pacillio, my mom Anna Cassella, and my father-in-law Frank Criscuolo, my brother-in-law Michael Criscuolo, Bill Molta, Sergio Gonzalez, Thimika Vega, and Claudia McCarthy, along with our other dedicated staff members continue to operate "my favorite restaurant" so well that I feel able to pursue my many other dreams. I can never thank them enough for their dedication to the high standards that we strive to maintain at **Claire's**.

Our wonderful customers continue to give us the positive energy it takes to run a successful restaurant, with their kind and considerate ways and their frequent smiles. I must also thank our vendors and our landlord for keeping up with our relentless pursuit of consistent quality.

Julia Moskin, my editor at Penguin, once again supported my work through her enthusiasm for the project, and by her direction she shaped a book that we can both be proud of. She and the entire editorial department really know how to make a good book even better—by challenging me to include important information that would have been easy for me to leave out. Many thanks to everyone at

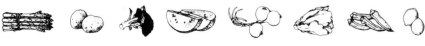

Penguin USA for their immeasurable help in production, promotion, and sales. A book is the result of a huge effort by many. I am also grateful to Carol Abel, my agent who takes care of an area I am least equipped to handle—contracts, legal terminology, and the other legal "stuff" that is vital to an author's success. I hope I never have to learn how to scrutinize a publishing contract!

Special thanks to my dear friend Louise Povinelli who helped to chop "way too many vegetables" and gave me the encouragement I needed, especially toward the end. When you write a cookbook, you naturally have a lot of leftover food around the house. My dear neighbors at The Windsor helped me by eating and complimenting the results of my work.

So many of the recipes that follow were inspired by or given to me by fellow Americans who, like me, love to celebrate our heritage through our foods. Special thanks to each person who shared their time and their recipes with me.

My cherished family and friends are always the greatest source of the energy that fuels my creativity. I hope I will always earn your love and support and bring you continued pride.

Frank, my partner in business and the love of my life, wears so many other hats. He is my sounding board ("Frank, what do you think about a little goat cheese in this?"), my friend, and my companion, but most important, he provides great love and balance in my life, and his wild sense of humor keeps me laughing, even after Julia Moskin called to ask if I can turn this book in six weeks early! I love being married to him.

Above all, I give thanks and praise to God.

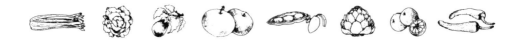

Contents

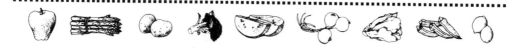

Introduction

When you are born into a family of marvelous cooks, your destiny is predetermined. I was brought up in a home where my brothers and I were spoiled with homemade eggnog and freshly squeezed orange juice at breakfast each day. We lived on Wooster Street in New Haven, Connecticut, a neighborhood of Italian immigrants. There were three apartments in our building and my grandfather's grocery store, Paolo Bigio and Sons, was on the ground level. Our apartment was over the store and next to my grandparents' apartment. My mother's brother Jimmy and his family lived in an apartment in our building, too, and my Uncle Bob, who remained a bachelor for many years, lived at home with my grandparents. Between my mom, her mom, and Uncle Jimmy's wife, Aunt Rose, there was always a pot of soup simmering on the stove. Freshly baked cream puffs, biscotti, and breads were waiting to be served with espresso, and platters of zucchini cutlets or eggplant Parmesan were always there for tasting. It didn't matter which apartment you entered; there was always something wonderful to eat.

With a loving grandmother, aunt, and mother all in the same house, I was always sure of getting someone to make my favorite foods. My standards for high-quality, delicious homemade food were firmly established by the time I reached the age of four. My mom says that I loved everything! I have to admit that little has changed regarding my love and respect for food.

When I was barely five years old, the New Haven Redevelopment Agency decided that Wooster Street would become the artery for a new highway. We left our beloved Italian neighborhood for the suburbs and for a new neighborhood where my mom said I would meet other "Americans." This move turned out to

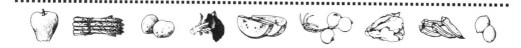

be a blessing in disguise. In our new neighborhood, I began to learn how other groups celebrated their heritage through their food traditions. In East Haven, we enjoyed Mary Funk's Hungarian goulash, Mrs. Garrity's Irish stews, Deborah Laurie's Jewish kugels, along with Mary Moniello's Italian pane cote. Life was delicious! My mom's great love for cooking and for experimenting with new recipes meant we could enjoy vegetarian versions of these newly discovered dishes on Fridays and Wednesdays, when our family, like most Italian Catholics, abstained from eating meat.

My experiences continued to expand when my older brother Billy took me to New York City to visit museums, art galleries, and restaurants. If you have any interest in eating fabulous food, and we certainly did, New York is the place to be! Because of the vast ethnic diversity of the city, I found a variety of cuisines unlike any other place I had ever visited.

By the early seventies, my brother Billy was spending his summers in Europe. He returned with photographs and vivid stories describing the foods he tasted. That is when my interest in foods grew from just eating to encompass cooking. I not only learned to make the dishes that I was familiar with, but I began to borrow cookbooks from the library (we didn't have any at home—*Claire's Corner Copia Cookbook* was the first cookbook that my mom ever owned) about Chinese and French cooking. My mom was a little disappointed that I was so interested in cooking that wasn't "Grandma's cooking," until I assured her that this was "someone else's grandmother's cooking."

In 1975, after graduating from college, I married Frank Criscuolo and together we opened **Claire's Corner Copia** intending to serve homemade foods from "everyone's grandmother." Our location across from Yale University gave me the opportunity to employ and meet people from all over the world. I loved it! Every day brought new ideas and recipes from our staff and our customers.

For the **Claire's** menu, I drew upon the many meatless dishes my mom cooked on Fridays and Wednesdays when I was growing up. Her creativity gave me lots of ideas about how to adapt recipes to a vegetarian diet. From my staff and customers, I also learned about the great vegetarian traditions of many world cuisines. There is the Italian vegetable soup *straciatella*, and a similar Chinese soup we call eggdrop. The Italian pasta dumplings that I knew as ravioli had delicious counterparts in Jewish kreplach, the Polish pierogi, and Asian wontons. Making these connections was both fascinating and delicious.

As our customers grew in both number and loyalty, we became the premier

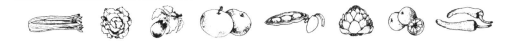

destination in Connecticut for a bounty of homemade vegetarian foods. **Claire's** grew and continues to thrive, even twenty years later.

After seventeen years as the executive chef, part owner, and general manager of **Claire's**, I had a wonderful opportunity to create what I considered to be an extension of the restaurant: *Claire's Corner Copia Cookbook*. This led to invitations to teach cooking classes across America. It's a joy to travel and meet fellow Americans who share my interest in cooking. I am thrilled to teach people how to make polenta, Sicilian rice balls, tamales, curries, and the many other vegetarian foods that I love. It is greatly rewarding to show someone who thinks they can't cook just how easy it is to prepare a fresh lentil vegetable soup or how to buy and cook broccoli rabe.

I learn so much from traveling. For example, I met people in San Antonio, Texas, who taught me how to make chicken-fried steaks. Then I taught them how to make chicken-fried veggie burgers. Many, many people have shared with me the ethnic and regional specialities they love. These healthful vegetarian versions are my return gift to all of them.

American diets are changing, and supermarkets across the country are responding to our growing demands for a greater selection of fresh vegetables, fruits, and other whole foods that may have originated in other countries but are now truly American. I have found fresh chilies in East Haven, Connecticut; fresh jicama in Evansville, Indiana; jasmine rice in Austin, Texas; broccoli rabe in St. Louis, Missouri; a plentiful supply of fresh cilantro in Nashville, Tennessee; and perfect squash blossoms in Boulder, Colorado.

Of course, as you'll see in the following recipes, Italian food is my first and greatest love. In my travels across the country, I've found that to be true of lots of people who aren't even Italian! Everyone especially loves pasta. Although my all-time favorite pasta sauce is a simple one of tomatoes, basil, and garlic made with good, extra-virgin olive oil and little else, I also love sauces made with vegetables, particularly meaty-textured mushrooms—and I do go in for an occasional rich cream sauce. I actually prefer cream sauces made with soy milk rather than with cream. The flavor is delicious yet light, and I don't feel bogged down after eating my Rigatoni with Mushrooms in a Creamy Whisky Sauce (page 160) the way I used to after a big plate of creamy pasta. And then there are the health benefits from eating soy foods to consider. In the following recipes, I'll show you how to make soy food a delicious addition to your daily diet.

Pastas, like any other food, vary in taste and quality. You should try a variety

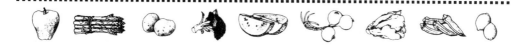

until you find the brands that best suit your tastes. The same rule applies to canned tomatoes and olive oils. When using canned tomatoes for my sauces, I always prefer Italian San Marzano tomatoes because of their superb quality, silky texture, and sweet flavor. When I find them I usually buy them by the case.

I always use extra-virgin olive oil, particularly from Sicily, for my sauces and salads and for many of my vegetable dishes, too. In fact, I often use extra-virgin olive oil to replace standard quality olive oil. Fortunately, the flavor of a good extra-virgin olive oil is so intense that you can use less of it, which will help to offset the added expense to both your pocket and your calories.

What started out as ethnic food is now becoming classic American food. Of course, you don't have to be Italian to love pasta, or of Spanish descent to enjoy a beautiful paella. You only need to be ready and willing to try these and the many other marvelous dishes that make our cuisine so special and diverse. I hope you enjoy eating your way through this book of truly American foods.

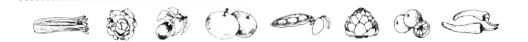

Glossary of Terms

I have included a short glossary of terms to describe ingredients that you might not be familiar with. Many of these foods are new here in America, but they have been healthful staples in Asian diets for centuries.

Tofu is a bean curd made from soybeans. It has a creamy color and little flavor of its own but quickly picks up the flavors of the foods it is cooked with. Tofu is rich in calcium, protein, and minerals, and is cholesterol-free, although soybeans do have a relatively high fat content. There are brands of fat-reduced tofu. Many researchers say tofu contains "good fat" and that soyfoods can lower cholesterol levels and possibly even reduce our chances of developing cancer. Tofu is found in the refrigerator section of most supermarkets, and you can buy it in aseptic packs (that don't require refrigeration) at most health food stores.

Tempeh is fermented soybeans with a firm texture and a rich, nutty, slightly smoky taste. You can find it in either the refrigerated or the freezer section of many supermarkets and in health food stores. Tempeh is rich in protein, calcium, and minerals. Avoid tempeh with black spots, which mean that it is past its prime, but white spots are fine and to be expected.

Soy Milk is made from soybeans and water or soy flour and water and is widely available in health food stores and supermarkets. It comes in aseptic packs that don't require any refrigeration until they are opened. Soy milk comes in flavors, usually plain, vanilla, carob, or chocolate, and is available in a range of fat content choices. I use plain soy milk in my cooking unless I specify otherwise (but I

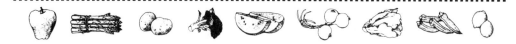

do love an occasional glass of cold, chocolate soy milk). Soy milk is lactose-free and gives you the health benefits of eating soy foods. It's great for making cream-style soups and pasta sauces.

Tofu Dogs, Meatless Hot Dogs, and Veggie Hot Dogs are found in health food stores and are also widely available in the freezer section of many supermarkets. Read the labels and decide just what you want to eat. Try several brands and choose your favorites. I usually test meatless hot dogs, burgers, and bacon on my nephew Branden—he loves the meat versions (although his parents try to keep them from his diet), and children are renowned for their honesty so he is a perfect judge. He has his favorites, which happen to be my favorites, too, and they are the brands I suggest in this book.

Meatless Sausage, Meatless Bacon, and Meatless Burgers are becoming quite the food trend. Worthington Foods has been in the business of manufacturing meatless foods for years, and they have recently launched the Morning Star Farms brand, a more natural line of meatless foods. Even Green Giant from Pillsbury is manufacturing a delicious vegetarian Harvest Burger. You can find meatless burgers and meatless versions of bacon and sausages in the freezer section of most supermarkets, but health food stores will usually have more natural products. I have indicated the brands that I used for specific recipes, but I encourage you to try as many as you can and then decide which are your favorites.

Spectrum Spread is the only nonhydrogenated butter alternative that I know of. It is made of 100% canola oil and you can buy it at your health food store. I use Spectrum to make biscuits and for other baking, and it makes a delicious spread for your toast. But don't try to sauté with it—it doesn't melt.

1
Soups

- Escarole, Potato, and Tomato Soup
- Polish Mushroom-Barley Soup
- Spinach and Pastina Soup
- Tomato Soup with "Sausage," Peppers, and Potatoes
- Asparagus Soup with Arborio Rice
- Mexican Pinto Bean and Vegetable Soup
- Split Pea Soup
- Risi e Fagioli (Italian Rice and Bean Soup)
- Creamy Asparagus Soup
- Soba Noodles with Chinese Cabbage in Broth
- Kidney Bean and Spinach Soup
- Garden Vegetable Soup with Chick-peas and Rice
- Straciatella
- Cabbage Borscht
- Thai Vegetable Soup
- Zucchini Soup with Arborio Rice
- Curried Potato, Corn, and Bell Pepper Soup
- Colcannon Soup
- Matzo Ball Soup
- Zucchini-Tomato Soup
- Cauliflower "Cream" Soup
- Tortilla Soup
- Sweet Potato and Corn Chowder
- Manhattan Vegetable Chowder

Escarole, Potato, and Tomato Soup

SERVES 8

Enjoy this traditional Italian soup for dinner with Cauliflower Pancakes (page 72) or Fresh Corn Polenta with Tomatoes and Basil Ricotta (page 115) and plenty of good bread for dunking.

4 tablespoons extra-virgin olive oil
6 large cloves garlic, minced
1 large onion, coarsely chopped
1 teaspoon crushed red pepper
2 large heads escarole, chopped into 1-inch pieces (see Note)
 Salt and black pepper
1 28-ounce can Italian peeled tomatoes, with juice, squeezed with your hands to crush
3 quarts water
1 teaspoon dried oregano
6 large potatoes, peeled and cut into 1½-inch cubes
 Salt and pepper

Heat the oil in a large soup pot over low to medium heat. Add the garlic, onions, and crushed red pepper. Cover and cook for 5 minutes, stirring occasionally, until the onions are softened, but not browned. Add the escarole. Sprinkle with salt and pepper. Stir to mix. Cover and continue cooking over low heat for 15 minutes, stirring occasionally, until the escarole is wilted and has released its juices.

Add the tomatoes, water, and oregano. Raise the heat to high. Cover and bring to a boil. Then reduce the heat to low to medium and continue cooking at a medium boil for 30 minutes, stirring occasionally. Add the potatoes. Cover and continue cooking for 40 minutes at a medium boil, stirring occasionally, until the potatoes are tender. Add salt and pepper to taste.

NOTE: Escarole can be gritty. I find it best to separate the leaves and soak them briefly in tepid water (I fill my sink), allowing any grit to sink to the bottom. Then I lift out the leaves, leaving the grit behind. Repeat the process in fresh water, if necessary.

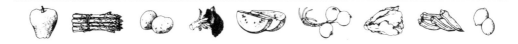

Polish Mushroom-Barley Soup

SERVES 8

This traditional Polish soup recipe was given to me by Charlie Skowronek, a former employee who is of Polish descent. My customers love all mushroom-barley soup but this one is their favorite.

4 tablespoons soybean margarine (found in health food stores) or butter
2 medium onions, coarsely chopped
2 large cloves garlic, minced
½ cup coarsely chopped fresh Italian flat-leaf parsley
4 medium carrots, coarsely chopped
4 ribs celery, cut into ¼-inch slices
½ medium head green cabbage, quartered, then coarsely chopped
3 quarts water
½ pound barley
1 bay leaf
1 tablespoon dried dillweed
2 potatoes, unpeeled, cut into ½-inch dice
1 pound mixed button and cremini mushrooms, cut into ¼-inch slices
3 cups low-fat plain yogurt
  Salt and pepper

Melt the margarine in a large soup pot over medium heat. Add the onions, garlic, parsley, carrots, celery, and cabbage. Cover and cook for 15 minutes, stirring occasionally, until the vegetables release some of their juices. Stir in the water. Cover and raise the heat to high. When the soup reaches a boil, stir in the barley and add the bay leaf. Lower the heat to medium and cook, covered, at a medium boil for about 1½ to 2 hours, stirring occasionally, until the barley is soft.

Stir in the dillweed, potatoes, and mushrooms. Cover and continue cooking for about 30 minutes, stirring frequently, until the potatoes are tender-soft. Place the yogurt in a large saucepan. Ladle about 2 cups of the hot soup into the yogurt and stir it to heat the yogurt. Pour the yogurt back into the soup. Stir it to combine. Lower the heat to low, and cook the soup for a minute or two, stirring continuously until it is heated through. Do not let the soup boil or the mixture will separate. Add salt and pepper to taste. Remove the bay leaf.

Spinach and Pastina Soup

SERVES 8

My New Haven grandmother was a big fan of spinach and of pastina, the tiny pasta stars so often used in Italian homemade soups. I was a big fan of hers and of everything she cooked. This healthy, oh-so-easy soup is no exception. Just be sure to get all the grit out of the spinach before cooking it.

    3 10-ounce bags fresh spinach
    4 tablespoons soybean margarine (found in health food stores) or butter
       Salt and pepper
    3 quarts water
    1½ cups uncooked pastina (tiny pasta stars)
       Freshly grated Romano cheese (optional)

Fill your sink with cool water. Open one bag of spinach at a time. Tear the leaves into small pieces then drop them into the water. When all of the spinach is in the water, swish the spinach around using your hands to loosen any sand from the leaves. Lift out handfuls of spinach into a large colander set in a bowl. Set aside to drain. Repeat until all the spinach is washed and completely free of grit.

Melt the margarine in a large soup pot over low heat. Add the spinach. Sprinkle with salt and pepper. Cover and cook over low heat for 15 minutes, stirring occasionally, until the spinach is wilted and has released all its liquids. Add the water. Raise the heat to high. Cover and bring to a boil, then reduce the heat to medium-low. Continue cooking, covered, at a medium boil for 30 minutes, stirring occasionally. Stir the pastina into the boiling soup. Raise the heat to medium-high. Continue cooking, uncovered, at a medium to rapid boil for 10 minutes, stirring frequently, until the pastina is tender and the soup is thickened. Taste for seasonings. Serve with grated Romano cheese and additional pepper on top, if desired.

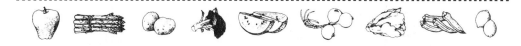

Tomato Soup with "Sausage," Peppers, and Potatoes

SERVES 8

This traditional southern Italian soup is as hearty as a stew. In fact, it is so satisfying that all you'll want (or need) is some good bread and perhaps a side dish of White Beans Stewed with Tomatoes and Sage (page 114) for a lovely dinner. I like Lean Links Sausage substitute by LightLife Foods.

2 tablespoons olive oil
5 large cloves garlic, finely chopped
4 medium yellow onions, coarsely chopped
4 large bell peppers (red, yellow, and/or green), seeded and coarsely chopped
  Salt and pepper
2 large fresh tomatoes, halved and cut into ½-inch wedges
1 35-ounce can Italian whole peeled tomatoes, with juice
4 cups water
3 large potatoes, peeled and cut into 1-inch chunks
1 tablespoon fennel seeds
1 large bay leaf
1 12-ounce package of meatless, Italian-style "sausage" (found in most health food stores), partially defrosted if frozen, cut into 1-inch pieces

Heat oil in a large soup pot over medium heat. Add the garlic, onions, and bell peppers. Sprinkle lightly with salt and pepper. Stir well to mix and coat evenly with oil. Cover and cook over medium heat for 10 to 12 minutes, stirring occasionally, until the vegetables have softened somewhat and have released some of their liquids. Add the fresh tomatoes, canned tomatoes and their juices, water, potatoes, fennel seeds, and bay leaf. Sprinkle lightly with salt and pepper. Stir well to mix. Raise the heat to high. Cover and bring to a full boil, then lower the heat to medium-low. Cover and cook at a low-medium boil for about 35 minutes, until the potatoes are just tender when tested with a fork. Stir occasionally. Break up any whole tomatoes with your spoon. Add the sausage, separating the pieces as you add them to the pot. Cover and continue cooking at a low-medium boil for 30 minutes, stirring occasionally. Taste for seasoning. Remove the bay leaf.

Asparagus Soup with Arborio Rice

SERVES 6

This is the soup that most reminds me of spring at my grandmother's house. We always enjoyed the tender young asparagus in a variety of dishes, including this traditional Italian soup thickened with arborio rice, the Italian short-grain rice also used in risottos. There was always a pot of this beautiful yet simple soup each spring, just waiting for Grandma to ladle us a bowlful. Then she would grate Parmesan or provolone cheese on top, and offer us good Italian bread for dunking.

  4 tablespoons soybean margarine (found in health food stores), or butter
  2 large sweet onions (preferably Vidalia), finely chopped
2½ pounds asparagus (about 2 bunches), tough bottoms removed, cut in ½-inch pieces
  1 teaspoon dried thyme
 ½ teaspoon dried sage
  1 bay leaf
  3 quarts water
    Salt and pepper
  1 cup arborio rice

Melt the margarine in a medium soup pot over low-medium heat. Add the chopped onions, cover, and cook for 10 minutes, stirring occasionally, until the onions are softened. Add the asparagus. Sprinkle with the thyme and sage. Add the bay leaf. Stir to mix. Cover and continue cooking for another 10 minutes, stirring occasionally. Add the water and sprinkle with salt and pepper. Stir to mix. Cover, raise the heat to high, and bring to a boil.

After the soup reaches a boil, reduce the heat to low and cook at a low-medium boil for 25 minutes, stirring occasionally. Stir in the arborio rice. Cover and continue cooking at a low-medium boil for about 45 minutes, stirring frequently, until the rice is tender and the broth is rich. Stir frequently or the rice will stick. Remove the bay leaf. Taste for seasonings.

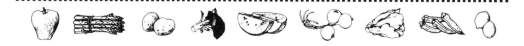

Mexican Pinto Bean and Vegetable Soup

SERVES 8

Javier Lopez, one of our shining stars at **Claire's**, *hails from Chihuahua, Mexico, and his culinary abilities and preferences have influenced us all. He introduced us to the delicious, delicate flavor of the popular Mexican pinto bean.*

12 ounces (about 1¾ cups) pinto beans, picked over for stones
 3 quarts water
 3 tablespoons olive oil
 2 medium yellow onions, coarsely chopped
 ¼ cup coarsely chopped fresh Italian flat-leaf parsley
 ¼ cup coarsely chopped fresh cilantro
 2 teaspoons chili powder
 2 teaspoons cumin
 1 small jalapeño pepper, stemmed and finely chopped (wash your hands immediately after handling hot peppers)
 4 medium carrots, peeled and cut into ¼-inch slices
 4 ribs celery, including leaves, cut into ¼-inch slices
 2 medium zucchini, cut in half lengthwise, then into ¼-inch slices
 1 medium sweet potato, peeled, cut in quarters lengthwise, then into ¼-inch slices
   Fresh corn kernels cut from 3 large ears of corn (about 3 cups), *or*
   2 10-ounce packages frozen kernels
   Salt and pepper

Put the pinto beans and the water in a large soup pot. Cover and bring to a boil over high heat. Lower the heat to medium. Stir in the olive oil, onions, parsley, cilantro, chili powder, cumin, and jalapeño pepper. Cover and cook at a medium boil for 45 minutes, stirring occasionally. Add the carrots and celery. Cover and continue cooking for 45 minutes, stirring occasionally, until the beans are just tender.

Stir in the zucchini and sweet potatoes. Cover and continue cooking for about 30 minutes. Stir in the corn, and salt and pepper to taste. Cover and continue cooking for 5 minutes, stirring occasionally. Taste for seasonings.

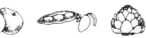

Split Pea Soup

SERVES 8

This is one of my most treasured recipes, passed down from my grandmother to my mother, to me, and now to you. Please pass it on to your loved ones.

½ stick (4 tablespoons) soybean margarine (found in health food stores) or canola oil
2 medium onions, coarsely chopped
4 quarts water
1 pound (2 cups) green split peas, picked over for stones
6 medium carrots, peeled and cut into ½-inch pieces
4 ribs celery, cut into ¼-inch pieces
2 large cloves garlic, minced
¼ cup finely chopped fresh Italian flat-leaf parsley
1 teaspoon dried basil
1 bay leaf
½ pound spaghetti, broken into 1-inch pieces
  Salt and pepper

Melt the margarine or heat the oil in a large soup pot over medium heat. Add the onions. Cover and cook for 10 minutes, stirring occasionally, until they are softened. Add the water. Cover and raise the heat to high. When it comes to a boil, add the split peas, carrots, celery, garlic, parsley, basil, and bay leaf. Stir well to mix. Cover and return to a boil, then lower the heat to low-medium. Cook, covered, at a low-medium boil, stirring occasionally, for 45 minutes. Remove the cover and raise the heat to medium. Cook at a medium boil for 1 hour, stirring occasionally, until the peas and vegetables are soft.

Stir in the broken spaghetti. Continue cooking for about 20 minutes, stirring occasionally, until the pasta is tender. Stir in salt and pepper to taste. Remove the bay leaf.

Risi e Fagioli
(Italian Rice and Bean Soup)

SERVES 8

If you like pasta e fagioli, an Italian favorite of pasta and beans cooked in a tomato sauce, then you'll love this recipe. The flavor is delicious and becomes even more so with freshly grated Romano cheese and additional black pepper on top. Add some good Italian bread (spread peanut butter on top for a surprisingly tasty treat) and a simple tossed salad and you may not want anything else for dinner—except a second bowlful.

    4 quarts water
    1 pound (2 cups) Roman, cranberry, or other pink beans, picked over for stones
    4 bay leaves
    6 large cloves garlic, thinly sliced
    3 ribs of celery with leaves, finely chopped
    1 small onion, finely chopped
    ¼ cup plus 2 tablespoons extra-virgin olive oil
    ¼ cup chopped fresh Italian flat-leaf parsley
    1 6-ounce can tomato paste
    1 medium tomato, chopped (juices included)
      Salt and pepper
    4 cups cooked brown or white rice

Place water, beans, and bay leaves in a large covered soup pot. Bring to a boil over high heat, then lower heat to medium. Cook, covered, at a low to medium boil for 1 hour, stirring only once, after about 30 minutes. Add garlic, celery, onion, ¼ cup of the olive oil, parsley, tomato paste, and the tomato. Raise heat to high, cover, and return to a full boil (this should take only a few minutes), then lower heat to medium. Cook, covered, at a medium boil for 1¼ hours, until the beans are nearly tender, stirring occasionally. Stir in the remaining 2 tablespoons of olive oil, and salt and pepper to taste. Continue cooking, uncovered, at a medium boil, for about 30 minutes, stirring occasionally, until the beans are tendersoft and the broth is creamy. Stir in the cooked rice. Cook until heated through. Taste for seasonings. Remove the bay leaves.

Creamy Asparagus Soup

SERVES 6

This beautiful dairy-free soup is made with asparagus, leeks, potatoes, and corn. It has all of the full, rich flavor of classic cream soups—with none of the cholesterol or the guilt.

3 tablespoons canola oil
1 large leek, chopped (wash carefully, they have loads of sand)
2 pounds asparagus (about 2 bunches), tough bottoms removed, cut in ½-inch pieces
2 large potatoes, peeled and chopped
   Fresh corn kernels cut from 3 to 4 large ears of corn (about 3½ cups), *or* 2 10-ounce packages frozen kernels
1 shallot, minced
⅛ teaspoon nutmeg
5 cups water
4 cups soy-rice milk (found in health food stores and some supermarkets)
1 tablespoon flour
   Salt and pepper

Heat the canola oil in a medium soup pot over low-medium heat. Add the leek, asparagus, potatoes, corn, shallot, and nutmeg. Cover and cook for 15 minutes, stirring occasionally. Add the water. Place 2 cups of the soy-rice milk in a blender. Add the flour, cover, and blend at high speed for 15 seconds. Pour this and the remaining 2 cups of soy-rice milk into the soup. Stir well to combine. Cover and raise the heat to high. Bring to a boil.

Lower the heat to medium and cook at a low-medium boil for about 25 minutes, stirring occasionally, until the asparagus are tender. Purée the soup, either moving a hand-blender around in the pot for about 2 minutes, or blending half cupfuls at a time on the low speed of your blender for 1 to 2 minutes until lightly puréed, stopping every 10 seconds or so to scrape down the sides of the blender cup. Add salt and pepper to taste.

NOTE: If you are using a blender, please be careful not burn yourself—hot liquid expands, rising up in the blender, and if the blender cup is more than half-filled, the hot soup will leap out of the cup and might burn your hand.

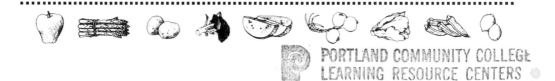

Soba Noodles with Chinese Cabbage in Broth

SERVES 4

You can buy soba, Asian buckwheat noodles, at health food stores. My favorite kind are made with wild yam flour—yams are so good for us, with their high content of beta-carotene. This soup, served with Stir-Fried Asian Vegetables (page 98), will make a terrific light supper.

2 tablespoons peanut oil
2 bunches scallion (about 10), white part and 3 inches of green, finely chopped
1 head Chinese cabbage (about 2 pounds), finely shredded
1 tablespoon finely minced, peeled gingerroot
½ teaspoon ground chili paste *or* ½ teaspoon crushed red pepper plus
    ¼ teaspoon ground red pepper (cayenne)
1 8.8-ounce package soba noodles
2 cups water
1 tablespoon rice vinegar
¾ cup soy sauce
1 tablespoon honey
    Pepper (optional)

Heat the peanut oil in a large skillet over medium heat. Add the scallion, cabbage, ginger, and chili paste. Cover and cook for 15 minutes, turning the cabbage as it shrinks down.

Meanwhile, cook the noodles according to package directions. Reserve 1¼ cups of cooking liquid and drain the noodles. Return the noodles to the pot and pour the reserved cooking liquid over the noodles. Cover and set aside.

After the cabbage shrinks down (about 15 minutes), stir in the water, rice vinegar, soy sauce, and honey. Raise the heat to high. Cover and bring to a boil. When it reaches a full boil, lower the heat to low-medium. Cover and cook at a low-medium boil for 10 minutes, stirring occasionally. Turn this mixture into the pot of noodles. Continue cooking over low-medium heat for 15 minutes, stirring occasionally. Taste for seasonings. Add pepper, if desired.

Kidney Bean
and Spinach Soup

SERVES 8

Although red kidney beans are best known as a key ingredient in chili and in Latin red bean and rice dishes, they are also popular in Italian dishes such as minestrone or escarole and bean soup. The combination of fiber- and protein-rich kidney beans with iron- and vitamin-packed spinach makes this soup a healthy and flavorful choice.

    12 ounces (1½ cups) red kidney beans, picked over for stones
     3 quarts water
    ¼ cup extra-virgin olive oil
     4 large cloves garlic, finely chopped
    ¼ cup finely chopped fresh Italian flat-leaf parsley
     1 bay leaf
     1 28-ounce can Italian whole peeled tomatoes with juice, squeezed with
        your hands to crush
     2 10-ounce bags spinach, washed well and coarsely chopped
    ½ pound small pasta shells or elbows, cooked according to package directions
        Salt and pepper

Bring the beans and the water to a boil in a large covered soup pot over high heat. Lower the heat to medium. Cover and cook at a medium-high boil for 1 hour, stirring occasionally. Stir in the olive oil, garlic, parsley, bay leaf, and tomatoes. Cover and bring to a boil over medium heat (about 25 minutes). Cook, covered, at a medium boil for another hour, stirring occasionally until the beans are soft-tender.

Stir in the spinach. Continue cooking, covered, for 25 minutes, stirring frequently until the spinach is tender. Remove the bay leaf. Stir in the cooked pasta. Season with salt and pepper.

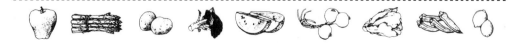

Garden Vegetable Soup with Chick-peas and Rice

SERVES 8

My mother cultivated our love for homemade soups by preparing a different one every day while we were growing up. My brothers and I still enjoy a bowl of soup for lunch or with dinner nearly every day. This soup resembles the Italian vegetable soups that my mom made toward the end of the week, using the vegetables that remained in the vegetable bin on the day before grocery day. Leftovers freeze well for up to a month. Why not make an extra batch for another day, or share your soup with others—friends and family just love the treat!

¼ cup plus 2 tablespoons extra-virgin olive oil
1 large sweet onion, chopped
3 quarts plus 1 cup water
4 medium carrots, peeled and coarsely chopped
4 ribs celery with leaves, cut into ⅓-inch slices
¼ cup chopped fresh Italian flat-leaf parsley
½ small head green cabbage, cored and chopped
½ small head cauliflower, cored and chopped
1 small butternut squash, peeled, seeded, and cut into ½-inch pieces
¼ pound string beans, cut into 1-inch pieces (about 1½ cups)
3 medium tomatoes, chopped
2 small sweet potatoes, peeled and cut into 1-inch cubes
2 small white potatoes, peeled and cut into 1-inch cubes
1 tablespoon salt
Pepper
1 tablespoon dried thyme
Fresh corn kernels cut from 2 to 3 large ears of corn (about 1½ cups), *or* 1 10-ounce package frozen kernels
½ cup frozen green peas
2 cups cooked or canned chick-peas
1½ cups cooked brown rice

    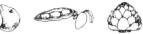

Heat ¼ cup of the olive oil in a large soup pot over low heat. Add the onions. Cover and cook slowly for 15 minutes, stirring occasionally, until the onions are soft and have released their juices. Add 1 cup of the water. Raise the heat to medium and cook for 15 minutes, stirring occasionally. Add the carrots, celery, parsley, cabbage, cauliflower, butternut squash, string beans, tomatoes, and sweet and white potatoes. Add the salt, pepper, and thyme. Add the remaining 3 quarts of water. Stir well to mix. Cover and raise the heat to high. When the soup reaches a full boil, remove the cover and lower the heat to medium.

Cook, uncovered, at a low-medium boil for 1 hour, stirring frequently until the soup looks creamy. Stir in the corn, green peas, chick-peas, and rice. Add the remaining 2 tablespoons of olive oil. Continue cooking at a low-medium boil for 30 to 45 minutes, stirring occasionally, until the vegetables are soft and the soup is thickened. Taste for seasonings.

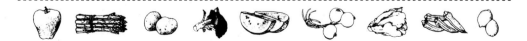

Straciatella

SERVES 8

There is no soup that reminds me of my beloved grandmother as much as this classic Italian soup. The aroma that fills my kitchen when I make this delicious vegetarian version transports me back to Grandma's kitchen. You can use dairy-free Parmesan, found in health food stores. I buy Soymage brand.

- 3 tablespoons soybean margarine (found in health food stores) or butter
- 1 large leek, white part and 3 inches of green, chopped
- 1 medium sweet onion, finely chopped
- 1 teaspoon dried thyme
- 1 teaspoon dried sage
- 1 bay leaf
- 5 large ribs of celery, finely chopped
- 3 medium carrots, peeled and finely chopped
- ½ cup chopped fresh Italian flat-leaf parsley
- ¼ cup chopped fresh basil leaves (or 2 tablespoons dried)
  Salt and pepper
- 3 quarts plus 1 cup water
- ¼ cup arborio rice
- 2 pounds fresh spinach, coarsely chopped
- 6 eggs or equivalent egg substitute
- ¼ cup grated Parmesan cheese

Melt the margarine in a large soup pot over low heat. Add the leek and onion. Sprinkle with the thyme and sage. Add the bay leaf. Cover and cook for 10 minutes, stirring occasionally. Add the celery, carrots, parsley, and basil. Add salt and pepper. Add the water. Raise the heat to high. Cover and bring to a boil. Decrease the heat to low. Cook, covered, at a low boil for 35 minutes, stirring occasionally. Stir in the rice and the spinach. Cover and continue cooking at a low boil for about 30 minutes, stirring frequently, until rice is just tender.

In a medium-size bowl, whisk together the eggs and the Parmesan cheese. Whisk in some additional pepper. Pour this slowly into the boiling soup. Stir well to combine. Cook for 5 minutes, stirring frequently. Taste for seasonings. Remove the bay leaf.

Cabbage Borscht

SERVES 8

*Many years ago, Norma Grannoff, the wife of our produce supplier at **Claire's**, shared her traditional Russian stuffed cabbage recipe with me. The savory sauce of her stuffed cabbage inspired this sweet and sour soup. Top each bowl with a dollop of sour cream and some finely chopped raw onion, and have plenty of good rye bread on hand for a lovely meal. Serve this flavorful soup with Russian Potato Salad (page 60) for a complete Russian-style meal.*

  2 tablespoons olive oil
  2 tablespoons soybean margarine (found in health food stores), or butter
  3 medium onions, cut in half, then thinly sliced
1½ large heads green cabbage, cored, cut in half, then thinly sliced
  1 medium potato, peeled and cut into ¼-inch pieces
  1 35-ounce can peeled tomatoes, with juice, squeezed with your hands to crush
  2 tablespoons tomato paste
  2 quarts water
  2 large lemons, squeezed, about ½ cup juice
  5 tablespoons sugar
    Salt and pepper

Heat the olive oil and margarine in a large soup pot over low-medium heat. Add the onions and cabbage. Cover and cook for 20 minutes, stirring occasionally, until the vegetables are softened and have released some of their liquids. Add the potato, tomatoes, tomato paste, and water. Stir well to mix. Cover, raise the heat to high and bring to a boil. When it comes to a boil, lower the heat to medium-low. Cook, covered, at a medium boil for 1 hour, stirring occasionally, until the cabbage and the potato are tender-soft.

Stir in the lemon juice and sugar. Cover and cook for 5 minutes, stirring occasionally. Stir in salt and pepper to taste.

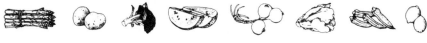

Thai Vegetable Soup

SERVES 6

This soup is flavored with lemongrass, but fresh lemongrass is not easy to come by. You need to have access to an Asian market, or to a produce manager who is willing and able to order it for you. For this recipe I use dried lemongrass, found in the spice section of most supermarkets, and although the flavor is not the same as fresh lemongrass, it still produces a delicious soup.

- 3 tablespoons peanut oil
- 4 large cloves garlic, minced
- 4 large ripe tomatoes, coarsely chopped, juices included
- ¼ cup finely chopped fresh cilantro
- 1-inch piece fresh ginger, peeled and minced
- 2 tablespoons ground chili paste (found in the condiment section of most supermarkets) or chopped fresh hot peppers
- 3 quarts water
- 2 large bell peppers (red and/or green), seeded and coarsely chopped
- 3 limes, squeezed, about 6 tablespoons juice
- 1 tablespoon dried lemongrass, ground with a mortar and pestle
- 2 zucchini, cut in ¼-inch slices
- 6 scallions, white part and 4 inches of green, cut into ¼-inch slices
- 6 button mushrooms, thinly sliced
- 12 snow peas, trimmed, cut into thirds
- Salt and pepper

Heat the oil in a large soup pot over medium heat. Add the garlic, tomatoes, cilantro, and ginger. Cover and cook for 5 minutes, stirring occasionally, until the tomatoes have released some of their liquids. Add the chili paste, water, bell peppers, lime juice, and lemongrass. Raise the heat to high. Cover and bring to a boil. Lower the heat to medium and cook at a medium-high boil for 45 minutes, stirring occasionally.

Add the zucchini, scallions, mushrooms, snow peas, and salt and pepper to taste. Cover and continue cooking at a medium boil for 30 minutes, stirring occasionally, until the zucchini are tender. Taste for seasonings.

Zucchini Soup with Arborio Rice

SERVES 8

This delicious Italian soup is made with zucchini and potatoes, with tomato paste added for a rich flavor. The arborio rice adds a creamy and luscious flavor without adding any cholesterol. It can be found either in the international section of your supermarket or near the other kinds of rice.

  3 tablespoons extra-virgin olive oil
  1 large clove garlic, minced
  2 medium onions, chopped
  3 large potatoes, cut into 1-inch cubes
 10 medium zucchini, cut into ½-inch slices
    Salt and pepper
  3 quarts water
  1 6-ounce can tomato paste
 ¼ cup chopped fresh Italian flat-leaf parsley
 ½ cup chopped fresh basil leaves
  1 cup arborio rice
    Freshly grated Romano cheese (optional)

Heat oil in a large soup pot over low heat. Add garlic and onions. Stir to coat with oil. Cover and cook for 10 minutes, stirring occasionally. Add the potatoes and zucchini. Add salt and pepper to taste. Stir to combine. Cover and continue cooking over low heat for 15 minutes, stirring occasionally. Add the water, tomato paste, parsley, and basil. Stir well to mix. Cover and raise the heat to medium-high. Bring the soup to a boil then reduce heat to low-medium. Cover and continue cooking at a low to medium boil for 45 minutes, stirring occasionally.

Add the rice and stir well to mix. Reduce the heat to low. Cover and continue cooking at a low boil for 25 minutes, stirring frequently (or the rice will stick), until the rice is tender. Taste for seasonings. Serve with freshly ground black pepper and grated Romano cheese on top, if desired.

Curried Potato, Corn, and Bell Pepper Soup

SERVES 8

This soup has a delicate curry flavor and a chunky combination of potatoes, corn, and bell peppers that everyone will love.

- 4 tablespoons soybean margarine (found in health food stores) or canola oil
- 3 medium onions, coarsely chopped
- 3 large cloves garlic, minced
- 2 large green bell peppers, seeded and coarsely chopped
- 6 large potatoes, peeled, cut in half lengthwise, then into thirds
- 1 tablespoon curry powder
- ½ cup finely chopped fresh Italian flat-leaf parsley
- 3 quarts water
- 1 bay leaf
  Fresh corn kernels cut from 3 large ears of corn (about 3 cups), *or* 2 10-ounce packages frozen kernels
- ¼ cup mango chutney
- 3 cups soy milk
- ¼ cup flour
  Salt and pepper

Melt the margarine or heat the canola oil in a large soup pot over medium heat. Add the onions, garlic, and bell peppers. Cover and cook for 5 minutes, stirring occasionally, until the onions have released some of their liquids. Add the potatoes, curry powder, and parsley. Stir to coat the potatoes. Stir in the water and bay leaf. Cover and raise the heat to high. Bring to a boil, then lower the heat to medium. Cook, covered, at a medium-high boil for 45 minutes, stirring occasionally, until the potatoes are soft and falling apart (this will thicken the soup).

Add the corn kernels and the chutney. Cover and continue cooking for 10 minutes, stirring occasionally. In a bowl, whisk together the soy milk and the flour until smooth. Slowly but steadily, pour the soy milk into the soup, stirring continuously. Cover and cook for 10 minutes, stirring frequently, until the soup is heated through and has thickened slightly. Remove the bay leaf. Taste for seasonings.

    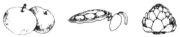

Colcannon Soup

SERVES 8

This is my soup version of the traditional Irish St. Patrick's Day favorite. But why wait for a holiday? Kale, cabbage, leeks, and potatoes make a wonderfully hearty and healthy soup any time you want to enjoy the delicious flavors of these Irish staples. Try it with a slice of good rye bread spread with spicy brown mustard.

- 2 pounds kale (about 2 large bunches)
- 2 tablespoons soybean margarine (found in health food stores) or canola oil
- 2 tablespoons olive oil
- 2 large leeks, white and 4 inches of green, coarsely chopped
- 1 large head savoy green cabbage (the kind with crinkly leaves), cored and finely chopped
  Salt and pepper
- 4 quarts water
- 6 large Idaho potatoes, peeled and chopped into 1-inch cubes
- 1 12-ounce package tofu hot dogs or other meatless hot dogs, cut into ½-inch pieces (found in most supermarkets and all health food stores)

Remove tough bottom stems from kale and discard. Chop the remaining leaves into 1-inch pieces. Melt the margarine or heat the canola oil with the olive oil in an extra-large soup pot over low heat. Add the kale, leeks, and cabbage. Add salt and pepper to taste and cover. After about 10 minutes, when the vegetables shrink down a little, stir to mix, using a long wooden spoon. Cover and cook for 25 minutes, stirring occasionally, until the vegetables are limp and have released their liquids.

Stir in the water. Raise the heat to high. Cover and bring to a boil (this should take about 20 minutes), then lower the heat to low-medium. Cover and cook at a medium boil, stirring occasionally, for an additional 35 minutes until the vegetables are tender. Taste and add a little more salt and pepper if needed. Add the potatoes, raise the heat to high and bring the soup back to a boil. Then lower the heat to low-medium and continue cooking, covered, at a medium boil for 15 to 20 minutes, stirring occasionally, until the potatoes are tender. Stir in the tofu hot dogs. Turn off the heat. Wait 2 minutes. Taste for seasonings.

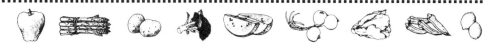

Matzo Ball Soup

SERVES 8

My friend Sheila Wolf introduced me to matzo ball soup, the quintessential Jewish cure-all, back in the early seventies. I immediately fell in love with the plump dumplings that are made from matzo, the unleavened bread eaten during the Jewish holiday of Passover. I couldn't let this beautiful chicken soup fall by the wayside when I adopted a vegetarian diet, so I began to experiment. My determination paid off. This matzo ball soup has a soft and delicately flavored matzo ball in each bowlful, and tender egg noodles floating in an herb-scented vegetable broth. Enjoy it with slices of dark rye bread spread with grainy mustard and Sweet and Sour Red Cabbage (page 89) for a delicious supper.

- 3 quarts water
- 2 medium onions, chopped
- 2 medium parsnips, peeled and chopped
- 4 medium carrots, peeled and chopped
- 8 large ribs celery with leaves, chopped
- 3 tablespoons soybean margarine (found in health food stores) or butter
- 1 tablespoon dried sage
- ¼ cup minced fresh Italian flat-leaf parsley
- 2 bay leaves
  Salt and pepper

Matzo Balls:

- ⅓ cup melted vegetable shortening
- 4 eggs or equivalent egg substitute
- 2 tablespoons minced fresh Italian flat-leaf parsley
- ½ cup water
- 1 cup matzo meal (found in the import or kosher section of most supermarkets)
- 4 ounces wide egg noodles, cooked according to package directions

Place the 3 quarts of water, onions, parsnips, carrots, celery, margarine, sage, parsley, and bay leaves in a large soup pot over high heat. Add salt and pepper to

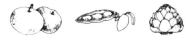

taste. Cover the pot and bring to a full boil, then lower the heat to low. Cook at a low boil for 2 hours, stirring occasionally, until the vegetables are soft. Remove the bay leaves. Taste for seasonings.

Meanwhile, prepare the matzo balls: In a bowl, whisk together the melted shortening, eggs, parsley, and water until blended. Stir in the matzo meal, mixing well to combine. Cover and refrigerate for 45 minutes to an hour until the batter is firm enough to form into balls. Roll the batter into balls the size of walnuts, placing them in a single layer on a platter or cookie sheet until you've used up all of the batter. After the soup has cooked for 2 hours, drop the matzo balls, one at a time, into the slowly boiling soup. Cook for 20 minutes, stirring gently after 15 minutes but not before or they will break up. Stir in the cooked egg noodles. Serve immediately.

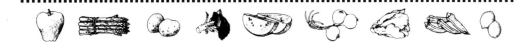

Zucchini-Tomato Soup

SERVES 8

What started out as an Italian soup, made to help use up each summer's abundant supply of zucchini, is now a pleasure-filled soup that we enjoy year-round.

3 tablespoons extra-virgin olive oil
2 medium onions, finely chopped
2 medium cloves garlic, minced
1 medium shallot, minced
1 rib celery with leaves, finely chopped
   Salt
1 28-ounce can whole tomatoes, with juice, squeezed with your hands to crush
¼ cup coarsely chopped fresh Italian flat-leaf parsley
¼ cup tomato paste
2 quarts water
1 bay leaf
2 teaspoons dried oregano
1 teaspoon dried basil
2 medium potatoes, peeled and diced into ½-inch cubes
5 medium zucchini, cut into ⅓-inch slices
6 medium button mushrooms, sliced
1 cup cooked or canned chick-peas
   Pepper

Heat oil in a medium soup pot over medium heat. Add the onions, garlic, shallot, and celery. Sprinkle lightly with salt. Cover and cook for 10 minutes, stirring occasionally, until the onions are softened. Add the tomatoes, parsley, tomato paste, and water. Cover the pot, raise the heat to high, and bring to a boil. Lower the heat to medium. Add the bay leaf, oregano, and basil. Cover and cook at a medium boil for 1 hour, stirring occasionally.

Add the potatoes, zucchini, and mushrooms. Raise the heat to high. Uncover and bring to a boil. Lower the heat to medium and cook, uncovered, at a low-medium boil for 1 hour, stirring occasionally, until the zucchini are soft-tender. Add the chick-peas, and salt and pepper to taste. Continue cooking, uncovered, for 5 minutes, stirring occasionally. Remove bay leaf. Taste for seasonings.

    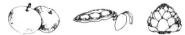

Cauliflower "Cream" Soup

SERVES 8

*There are many wonderful flavors in this soup, which combines cauliflower, pota-
toes, and a little tomato and dill to freshen the flavors in a rich and creamy broth.*

- ½ stick (4 tablespoons) soybean margarine (found in health food stores) or
  canola oil
- 1 large shallot, minced
- 1 medium sweet onion, minced
- 2 medium heads cauliflower, cored and finely chopped
- 4 medium potatoes, peeled and finely chopped
- ¼ cup finely chopped fresh Italian flat-leaf parsley
- 1 medium tomato, finely chopped, juices included
- 2 teaspoons dried dillweed
- 5 cups water
- 8 cups soy milk (found in most supermarkets and in health food stores)
- 4 tablespoons flour
  Salt and pepper

Melt the margarine or heat the canola oil in a large soup pot over medium
heat. Add the shallot, onion, cauliflower, potatoes, parsley, and tomato. Cover
and cook for 30 minutes, stirring occasionally until the vegetables are softened
and have released some of their liquids. Stir in the dillweed. Add the water and
raise the heat to high. Cover and bring to a boil. When it comes to a boil, lower
the heat to medium. Cover and cook at a medium boil for 1 hour, stirring occasionally until the vegetables are soft.

Using a potato masher, mash the vegetables in the soup pot. Measure the soy milk
into a bowl. Sift the flour over the soy milk, whisking in the flour as you sift. Whisk
until the flour is thoroughly mixed in. Gradually pour this mixture into the soup, stirring as you pour. Continue cooking, uncovered, for 20 minutes, stirring frequently
until the soup has thickened slightly and is fully heated. Stir in salt and pepper to taste.

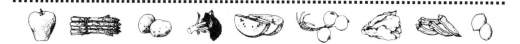

Tortilla Soup

SERVES 8

The fresh lime juice and cilantro give this popular Mexican soup its characteristic flavor. Serve it with warm corn tortillas—just tear the tortillas into small pieces and drop them right into your bowl. Serve with Avocado, Tomato, and Onion Salad (page 33) and Black Bean Quesadillas (page 242) for a delicious dinner.

4 tablespoons (½ stick) soybean margarine (found in health food stores) or canola oil
1 medium onion, finely chopped
4 ribs celery with leaves, coarsely chopped
2 large ripe tomatoes, finely chopped, juices included
2 medium parsnips, peeled and finely chopped
3 medium carrots, peeled and finely chopped
3 quarts water
2 teaspoons dried sage
1 bay leaf
¼ cup finely chopped fresh Italian flat-leaf parsley
½ cup finely chopped fresh cilantro
1 teaspoon chili powder
1 medium zucchini, finely chopped
2 scallions, white part and 4 inches of green, thinly sliced
2 limes, squeezed, about ½ cup juice
Salt and pepper
4 to 6 ounces shredded low-fat Monterey Jack cheese
4 corn tortillas, torn into fourths

Melt the margarine or heat the canola oil in a large soup pot over medium heat. Add the onion, celery, tomatoes, parsnips, and carrots. Cover and cook for 20 minutes, stirring occasionally, until the vegetables have released some of their liquids. Add the water, sage, bay leaf, parsley, cilantro, and chili powder. Raise the heat to high. Cover and bring to a boil. When it reaches a boil (in about 15 minutes), lower the heat to medium. Cook, covered, at a medium boil for 1 hour, stirring occasionally, until the parsnips are soft.

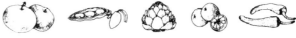

Add the zucchini, scallions, and lime juice. Cover and continue cooking for about 15 minutes, stirring occasionally, until the zucchini is tender. Season with salt and pepper. Taste for seasonings. Remove the bay leaf. Sprinkle a little shredded Monterey Jack in each bowl before filling with soup, then scatter a few pieces of tortilla over the top of each bowl.

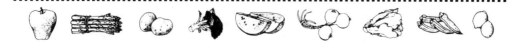

Sweet Potato and Corn Chowder

SERVES 8

My husband Frank and I make an annual trip to the seashore town of Gloucester, Massachusetts, where he enjoys the marvelous seafood chowders. This chowder is chunky with lots of fresh corn, plenty of sweet potato, and sweet onions. I have also added the traditional chowder flavoring of celery and the smokiness of meatless bacon.

  3 tablespoons soybean margarine (found in health food stores) or canola oil
  3 strips meatless bacon (found in health food stores), chopped
  1 large shallot, minced
  1 large sweet onion, finely chopped
  4 ribs celery, finely chopped
  1 tablespoon dried thyme
  1 bay leaf
    Salt and pepper
  ½ cup finely chopped fresh Italian flat-leaf parsley
  5 cups water
  5 large sweet potatoes, peeled and cut into 1-inch chunks
    Fresh corn kernels cut from 9 large ears of corn (about 9 cups) (see Note)
  7 cups soy milk
  2 tablespoons flour
  ½ teaspoon ground red pepper (cayenne)

Melt the margarine or heat the canola oil in a large soup pot over low-medium heat. Add the meatless bacon, shallot, onion, celery, thyme, and bay leaf. Sprinkle with salt and pepper to taste. Stir to mix. Cover and cook for 15 minutes stirring occasionally until the onion and celery soften. Add the parsley, water, and sweet potatoes. Stir to mix. Cover and raise the heat to medium. Bring to a low-medium boil. Cook, stirring occasionally, for 20 minutes or until the potatoes are barely fork-tender. Stir in the corn. Cover and continue cooking for about 10 minutes, stirring occasionally.

In a separate bowl whisk together the soy milk and the flour. Slowly pour this mixture into the soup, stirring continuously. Stir in the cayenne. Cover and continue cooking for about 10 minutes, stirring occasionally, until the soup is heated through and slightly thickened. Taste for seasonings. Remove the bay leaf.

NOTE: After you cut the kernels from the corn, scrape the bald cobs using the blade of your knife to squeeze out the corn liquid. Include this "cream" with your corn kernels.

Manhattan Vegetable Chowder

SERVES 8

Chowders are usually made with fish. This Manhattan variety is tomato-based with lots of chunky vegetables in a richly flavored broth.

- 2 tablespoons olive oil
- 1 tablespoon soybean margarine (found in health food stores) or butter
- 2 medium onions, minced
- 1 large clove garlic, minced
- 4 medium carrots, peeled and cut into ⅓-inch slices
- 4 large ribs celery with leaves, cut into ½-inch slices
- 4 medium potatoes, peeled and coarsely chopped
- ½ cup coarsely chopped fresh Italian flat-leaf parsley
- 1 tablespoon dried thyme
- 1 bay leaf
- 1 35-ounce can whole peeled tomatoes with juice, squeezed with your hands to crush
- 2 quarts water
- 2 tablespoons tomato paste
  Fresh corn kernels cut from 2 large ears of corn (about 2 cups), *or*
  1 10-ounce package frozen kernels
  Salt and pepper
- 3 to 4 dashes Tabasco

Heat the oil and margarine in a large soup pot over medium heat. Add the onions, garlic, carrots, celery, potatoes, and parsley. Cover and cook for 15 minutes, stirring occasionally, until the vegetables release some of their liquids. Add the thyme, bay leaf, tomatoes, water, and tomato paste. Raise the heat to high. Cover and bring to a boil. Lower the heat and cook, covered, at a medium boil for 1¼ hours, stirring occasionally, until the vegetables are soft-tender.

Stir in the corn, salt and pepper to taste, and the Tabasco sauce. Cover and continue cooking at a medium boil for 5 minutes, stirring occasionally. Remove the bay leaf. Taste for seasonings.

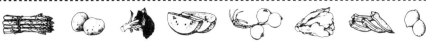

2
Salads and Dressings

- Avocado, Tomato, and Onion Salad
- Green Beans and Walnuts in a Creamy Garlic Dressing
- Jicama Salad
- Tuscan Salad of Chicory, White Beans, and Hearts of Palm
- Arugula, Tomato, and Goat Cheese Salad
- Green Bean Salad with Hearts of Palm and Pecans in a Creamy Orange-Tarragon Dressing
- Salad of Mixed Field Greens, Golden Raisins, and Goat Cheese
- Barley Salad
- Marinated Bean Salad with Oranges in an Orange Vinaigrette
- Southwestern Black Bean Salad with Chipotle-Lime Dressing
- Beet and Tofu Salad
- Fresh Corn Salad with Chipotle Vinaigrette
- Health Salad
- Mediterranean Orzo Salad
- Spanish Pasta Salad with White Beans and Vegetables
- Pasta Salad Copenhagen
- Pasta Salad with Asparagus and Pecans in a Citrus Vinaigrette
- Pasta Salad with Artichoke Hearts, Green Peas, and Hearts of Palm in a Creamy Garlic and Basil Dressing
- Waldorf Pasta Salad
- Summer Pasta Salad with Ricotta Cheese, Tomatoes, and Basil
- Fresh Tomato Salad

- Whole-Meal Salad with Granny Smith Apples and Tofu Hot Dogs in a Creamy Curry and Lime Dressing
- Russian Salad from Minsk
- Balsamic Vinaigrette
- Whole-Meal Potato Salad
- Pennsylvania Dutch Potato Salad
- Russian Potato Salad
- Sweet Potato Salad
- Italian Green Bean and Potato Salad
- French Potato Salad
- Creamy Tofu Salad with Grapes, Jicama, and Pecans
- Dairy-Free Green Goddess Dressing
- Dairy-Free Caesar Salad Dressing

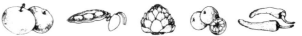

Avocado, Tomato, and Onion Salad

SERVES 6

The cilantro vinaigrette gives this salad a delicious Southwestern flavor. I like to serve warmed corn tortillas alongside. Toast the pine nuts in a skillet over medium heat just until light brown, watching them carefully to be sure they don't overcook.

    2 ripe avocados, peeled and cut into ½-inch cubes
    3 medium ripe tomatoes, cut in half then into ½-inch wedges
    1 small onion, finely chopped
    4 scallions, white part and 3 inches of green, cut into ¼-inch slices
    1 large clove garlic, minced
    ¼ cup sliced black olives
    ¼ cup toasted pine nuts
    3 tablespoons olive oil
    1 teaspoon finely grated lime zest
    2 limes, squeezed, about 3 tablespoons juice
    3 tablespoons minced fresh cilantro
      Salt and pepper

Place the avocados, tomatoes, onion, scallions, garlic, black olives, and pine nuts in a bowl. Gently toss to mix, using two spoons. Into a separate bowl, measure the olive oil, lime zest, lime juice, and cilantro. Whisk this together until well blended. Stir in salt and pepper to taste. Pour the dressing over the avocado salad and toss gently to coat the salad evenly. Taste for seasonings. Serve immediately or chilled.

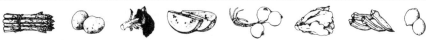

Green Beans and Walnuts in a Creamy Garlic Dressing

SERVES 8

Green beans taste so good and they can be used in a multitude of delicious ways, from soups to side dishes and luscious salads like this one.

- 1 pound green beans, trimmed
- ¾ cup soy milk (found in most supermarkets and in health food stores)
- 1 medium clove garlic, finely chopped
- ½ cup chopped fresh Italian flat-leaf parsley
- ¼ cup dairy-free mayonnaise (found in health food stores)
  Salt and pepper
- ½ head romaine lettuce, torn into large pieces
- ¼ cup chopped walnuts

Cook the green beans in lightly salted boiling water for about 5 minutes, or until crisp-tender to your preference. Drain well. Turn into a bowl. Measure the soy milk into a blender. Add the garlic, parsley, and mayonnaise. Cover and blend on high speed for 1 minute, until well blended. Stir in salt and pepper to taste. Pour the dressing over the green beans and toss well to mix, using two spoons. Arrange the torn romaine leaves on a large platter. Arrange the green beans over the romaine leaves and pour the dressing evenly over entire salad. Sprinkle the walnuts evenly over the top. Serve immediately.

Jicama Salad

SERVES 6

My first taste of this crunchy, sweet tuber from Mexico occurred in south Florida during the eighties. It was love at first bite! Jicama can be eaten either raw or cooked. It's terrific in stir-fries, too. It is beige, has a thin skin, and resembles a large turnip in shape. You can find it year-round in the produce section of most supermarkets. Buy a big one, use most of it for this salad, and save the other third to peel and eat as you would carrot sticks. I haven't yet met anyone who doesn't like its flavor. I use a paring knife to easily remove the skin from the jicama.

- 1 jicama (about 3 pounds), peeled and cut into 1-inch cubes
- 1 medium cucumber, peeled, seeded, and cut into 1-inch cubes
- 1 large Granny Smith apple, cut into ½-inch cubes
- 1 medium sweet onion (preferably Vidalia), sliced into thin rings
- 1 medium mango, peeled and cut into ½-inch cubes (don't worry if the cubes mash up a bit)
- ¼ cup chopped pecans
- 2 tablespoons olive oil
- 3 to 5 limes, squeezed, about 7 tablespoons juice
- 2 tablespoons chopped fresh cilantro
- 1 tablespoon grated orange zest
- Salt and pepper

Place all of the ingredients in a large mixing bowl. Toss well to mix, using two spoons. Taste for seasonings. Serve at room temperature or chilled.

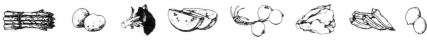

Tuscan Salad of Chicory, White Beans, and Hearts of Palm

SERVES 8

At La Trattoria, a wonderful Tuscan restaurant in Boca Raton, Florida, they make a salad that inspired this recipe. I had forgotten just how much I love the slightly bitter, almost lemon-peppery flavor of chicory with the delicate, distinctly artichoke-like flavor of hearts of palm. Hearts of palm are rather expensive, but they're so rich in calcium and iron and they taste so good that they are well worth the splurge. The gourmet or import sections of most supermarkets carry hearts of palm packed in cans or in jars.

    1 medium head chicory, cut into bite-size pieces
    1 head endive, cut into bite-size pieces
    1 small head radicchio, cut into bite-size pieces
    4 radishes, thinly sliced
    ½ small cucumber, peeled, seeded, and diced
    7 ounces canned hearts of palm, drained, cut into ¼-inch slices
    1 cup freshly cooked or canned drained white beans
    ½ small sweet onion, sliced thin
    2 large cloves garlic, minced
    3 tablespoons extra-virgin olive oil
    1 lemon, squeezed, about 4 tablespoons juice
      Salt and pepper

Place the chicory, endive, radicchio, radishes, cucumber, hearts of palm, beans, onion, and garlic in a large salad bowl. Toss well using two spoons. Drizzle the olive oil evenly over the salad. Toss to coat the leaves thoroughly. Drizzle the lemon juice over the salad. Toss well to mix evenly. Add salt and pepper to taste. Toss again to mix well.

Arugula, Tomato, and Goat Cheese Salad

SERVES 6

If you are fond of bitter greens like broccoli rabe, chances are you also like the assertive, slightly peppery taste of arugula. I've been hooked on arugula since my friend Jimmy Esposito first introduced me to this vitamin A- and C-packed traditional Italian green. In fact, my husband now grows arugula in our summer garden. Be sure to wash your arugula well, in several changes of water, until all of the fine sand is removed.

      3 tablespoons pine nuts
      2 large bunches arugula (about ¾ pound), well washed
  2½ tablespoons extra-virgin olive oil
      1 tablespoon balsamic vinegar
        Salt and pepper
      2 large ripe tomatoes, cut into ¼-inch slices
      1 clove garlic, minced
      4 ounces goat cheese, crumbled

Lightly toast the pine nuts in a skillet just until light brown. Set aside. Remove and discard the thick, tough stems from the arugula, but leave the thinner, tender stems on. Place the arugula in a large bowl. Add 2 tablespoons of the olive oil. Toss well. Add the balsamic vinegar, and salt and pepper to taste. Toss well. Arrange the arugula on a serving platter. Arrange the sliced tomatoes over the arugula. Scatter the minced garlic over the tomatoes. Sprinkle the tomatoes with salt and pepper. Scatter the crumbled goat cheese over the tomatoes. Drizzle the remaining ½ tablespoon olive oil over the tomatoes and goat cheese. Scatter the toasted pine nuts over the entire salad and serve.

Green Bean Salad with Hearts of Palm and Pecans in a Creamy Orange-Tarragon Dressing

SERVES 8

Hearts of palm are grown on the cabbage palm tree in tropical climates such as south Florida and Brazil. They have a flavor similar to artichokes, a delightful, creamy texture, and are fat-free. You can buy hearts of palm in cans or in jars, in the condiment or canned vegetable section of your supermarket.

- ¾ pound green beans, ends trimmed
- 1 7¾-ounce can hearts of palm, drained and cut into ¼-inch slices
- 4 tablespoons coarsely chopped pecans
- 2 medium tomatoes, each cut into ½-inch wedges

Dressing:

- ¾ cup soy-rice milk (found in health food stores and some supermarkets)
- ½ medium red (Bermuda) onion, coarsely chopped
- 1 juice orange, peeled and sliced, juices included
- 1 cup dairy-free mayonnaise (Nayonaise brand is found in health food stores), or low-fat mayonnaise
- 1 teaspoon dried tarragon
  Salt and pepper

Cook the green beans in about 5 cups of lightly salted boiling water for 5 to 7 minutes until crisp-tender. Drain. Run under cold water. Drain well. Turn into a bowl. Add the hearts of palm, pecans, and tomatoes. Toss gently to mix. Set aside while you prepare the dressing: Pour the soy-rice milk into a blender. Add the onion and the sliced orange with its juices. Cover and blend on low speed for 5 seconds, then raise the speed to high and continue blending for another 25 seconds. The mixture should have little pieces of the orange in the liquid. Turn into a bowl. Add the mayonnaise, tarragon, and salt and pepper to taste. Whisk well to mix. Pour over the salad. Toss gently to combine with two spoons. Taste for seasonings. Serve at room temperature or chilled.

Salad of Mixed Field Greens, Golden Raisins, and Goat Cheese

SERVES 6

We anxiously await summer for its beautiful blue skies and lovely, warm, sunny days—perfect days to enjoy a salad of tender, locally grown greens. This salad uses mesclun, a delicious blend of mixed baby lettuces, herbs, and edible flowers.

¾ pound mixed field greens (mesclun)
½ small sweet onion, thinly sliced
½ cup golden raisins
¼ cup slivered almonds
4 tablespoons extra-virgin olive oil
3 tablespoons balsamic vinegar
 Salt and freshly ground pepper
4 ounces goat cheese, broken into small pieces

Place the greens in a salad bowl. Add the onion, raisins, and almonds. Toss gently to mix. Sprinkle with the olive oil. Toss gently to coat the leaves. Sprinkle with the balsamic vinegar. Toss gently to mix. Sprinkle with salt and pepper to taste. Toss gently to combine. Taste for seasonings. Scatter pieces of goat cheese over the salad. Serve immediately.

Barley Salad

SERVES 8

Barley is a nice, nutty change from pasta or rice and is perfect in salads.

1 pound pearl barley
3 medium carrots, peeled and finely diced
2 cups broccoli florets
1 cup frozen green peas
½ cup golden raisins
1 large Granny Smith apple, cored and diced small
¼ cup extra-virgin olive oil
½ cup freshly squeezed orange juice
2 teaspoons dried tarragon
   Salt and pepper

Bring 4 quarts of lightly salted water to a boil in a large, covered pot over high heat. Add the barley, lower the heat to medium. Cook, covered, at a medium boil for about 1 hour, stirring occasionally, until the barley is tender. Stir in the carrots, broccoli florets, green peas, and raisins. Continue cooking for 2 minutes, stirring occasionally. Drain. Rinse under cold water and drain again. Turn into a bowl. Add the apple. Toss well using two spoons. In a separate bowl, whisk together the olive oil, orange juice, tarragon, and salt and pepper to taste. Pour the dressing over the salad and toss thoroughly to coat well. Taste for seasonings. Serve immediately or chilled.

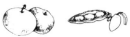

Marinated Bean Salad with Oranges in an Orange Vinaigrette

SERVES 8

My neighbor Lucy Bouck brought this vitamin C- and fiber-rich salad to one of our potluck cookouts and it was quite a hit. The combination of beans, onions, and orange juice is a delicious change from the usual 3-bean salads that we have all gotten used to over the years.

 1½ cups cooked red kidney beans
 1½ cups cooked great northern beans or other white beans
  1 cup cooked pinto beans
  1 medium red (Bermuda) onion, sliced into thin rings and separated
  1 small onion, sliced into thin rings and separated
  ¼ cup extra-virgin olive oil
  1 tablespoon finely grated orange zest
  ½ large orange, squeezed, about ½ cup juice
  1 tablespoon dry dillweed or 3 tablespoons chopped, fresh dill
    Salt and pepper

Place all of the ingredients into a bowl. Toss well to mix. Taste for seasonings.

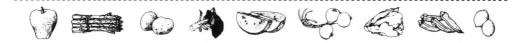

Southwestern Black Bean Salad with Chipotle-Lime Dressing

SERVES 8

Everyone loves this combination. The dressing gets its zip from the chipotle pepper and lime. Chipotle peppers are smoked jalapeños and are available dried in packages in the produce section of most supermarkets. Jicama is a tuber from Mexico and tastes like a combination of apple and water chestnut. Simply peel the skin and eat pieces of raw jicama as you would a fruit or vegetable, add it to a salad, or add it to stir fries.

Fresh corn kernels cut from 2 large ears of corn (about 2 cups),
   or 1½ 10-ounce packages frozen kernels
1 pound black beans, cooked according to package directions
4 scallions, white part and 3 inches of green, cut into ¼-inch slices
¼ medium jicama, peeled and cut into ¼-inch cubes
1 large red bell pepper, cut into ¼-inch pieces
1 medium tomato, cut into ½-inch cubes
1 medium-size ripe avocado, peeled and cut into ½-inch cubes

Dressing:

3 tablespoons water
1 small chipotle pepper
2 tablespoons olive oil
2 large limes, squeezed, about 5 tablespoons juice
1 teaspoon tequila
1 medium clove garlic, finely chopped
2 tablespoons chopped fresh cilantro or Italian flat-leaf parsley
1 cup soy milk
Salt and pepper

Cook the corn kernels in lightly salted, boiling water for 2 minutes. Drain and turn into a large bowl. Rinse the cooked black beans under cold water, drain well, then add them to the bowl with the corn. Add the scallions, jicama, bell pepper, tomato, and avocado. Toss gently but thoroughly.

Prepare the dressing: Bring the water to a boil in a small pot over high heat. Add the chipotle pepper. Cook for 2 minutes, turning frequently to cook evenly. Remove from the heat. Set aside until cool enough to handle. Meanwhile, measure the olive oil, lime juice, and tequila into a blender. Add the garlic and cilantro. When the chipotle pepper is cool enough to handle, remove and discard the stem. Coarsely chop it and add it with its juices and the cooking liquid to the blender. Cover and blend on high speed for 10 seconds. Stop and scrape down the sides using a rubber spatula. Cover and blend on high speed for 5 seconds, then, with the motor running, gradually add the soy milk. Continue blending for 10 seconds. Stir in salt and pepper to taste. Pour the dressing over the salad. Toss gently but thoroughly to mix. Taste for seasonings. Serve at room temperature or chilled.

Beet and Tofu Salad

SERVES 4

Every time I see a mound of beautiful, crimson red, fiber-rich beets at the market, my thoughts turn to this lovely, fresh salad. It's a perfect choice for a picnic or for a brown bag lunch because it travels so well. The flavors are so delicious that even those who think they don't like tofu will enjoy the zesty taste and the health benefits of this salad. Beets are fun to cook, too: The cooking water becomes an eye-catching pool of crimson. In fact, I've been tempted to lift the cooked beets from the pot, and then use the richly colored liquid as a dye for our white aprons at Claire's.

    3 large beets, peeled
    1 small red (Bermuda) onion, sliced into thin rings and separated
    1 pound firm or extra-firm tofu, drained and cut into ½-inch cubes
    ¼ cup olive oil
    ¼ cup red wine
    2 tablespoons balsamic vinegar
    ½ teaspoon dried oregano
      Salt and pepper

Cook beets in lightly salted boiling water for about 45 minutes, until just tender when tested with a fork. Drain. When cool enough to handle, slice beets in half, then slice each half into ¼-inch slices. Place in a bowl. Add the remaining ingredients. Toss gently to combine. Taste for seasonings. Serve immediately or chilled. Toss again just before serving.

Fresh Corn Salad with Chipotle Vinaigrette

SERVES 8

Chipotle peppers are smoked jalapeños. They are now readily available in most supermarkets, sold dried in small packages. I love the smoky, slightly hot flavor that chipotle peppers add to foods. They also give a nice zip to salad dressings, and work beautifully with all-American ingredients like corn and tomatoes.

Fresh corn kernels cut from 6 to 7 large ears of corn (about 6½ cups)
1 small zucchini, diced
3 large ripe tomatoes, diced
4 scallions, white part and 4 inches of green, cut into ⅛-inch slices
3 tablespoons olive oil
1 chipotle pepper
¼ cup water
2 limes, squeezed, about 3 tablespoons juice
3 tablespoons minced fresh cilantro
Salt and pepper

Bring 4 quarts of lightly salted water to a boil in a covered pot over high heat. Add the corn kernels. Cover and cook for 2 minutes until the corn is crisp-tender. Add the zucchini and cook for 1 minute. Drain. Turn into a bowl. Add the tomatoes and the scallions. Toss to mix, using two spoons.

Heat the olive oil in a medium pot over medium-high heat. Add the chipotle pepper. Cook the pepper for 3 minutes, turning frequently with tongs, to coat with oil. Add the water (it will sizzle slightly) and raise the heat to high. When the water comes to a boil, stir once then remove from the heat. Let the mixture cool for about 5 minutes, or until the pepper is cool enough to handle. Remove the stem from the pepper and discard. Chop the pepper finely. Return the chopped pepper and its juices to the pot. Stir in the lime juice, cilantro, and salt and (remember the chipotle pepper is hot) a little pepper to taste. Pour the dressing over the corn salad and toss thoroughly, using two spoons. Taste for seasonings. Serve at room temperature or chilled.

Health Salad

SERVES 8

This salad has many of my favorite foods in it—pasta, brown rice, beans, garlic, and tomatoes—and it is also a delicious way to use up those leftover portions of cooked beans and rice.

- 1 pound penne pasta
- 3 medium carrots, peeled and finely diced
- ½ cup cooked brown rice
- 1 cup cooked kidney beans
- 1 cup cooked or canned white beans
- ½ cup finely chopped fresh Italian flat-leaf parsley
- 4 medium cloves garlic, minced
- 2 medium ripe tomatoes, diced
- ¼ cup extra-virgin olive oil
   Salt and pepper

Cook the penne according to package directions, but stir in the carrots just before you drain the pasta. Drain the pasta and carrots. Rinse under cold water, then drain again. Turn the pasta and carrots into a large bowl. Add the brown rice, kidney beans, white beans, parsley, garlic, and tomatoes. Toss gently but thoroughly, using two spoons. Drizzle the olive oil evenly over the salad. Toss gently but thoroughly to coat the salad. Add salt and pepper to taste. Serve immediately or chilled.

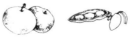

Mediterranean Orzo Salad

SERVES 6

I made my first orzo pasta salad in the early eighties when I was invited by the New Haven Register *to create a Labor Day picnic menu for a family of four on a budget of $12. The salad turned out to be very popular at* **Claire's** *and I've been making orzo pasta salads ever since.*

  1 pound orzo (rice-shaped) pasta
  2 large bell peppers (1 red and 1 yellow), stemmed, seeded, and finely chopped
  3 medium cloves garlic, minced
  1 10-ounce bag spinach, finely chopped
  1 medium red (Bermuda) onion, finely chopped
  1 large ripe tomato, diced
 12 to 18 calamata olives, pitted and halved
  3 tablespoons tiny capers, drained
  ¼ cup extra-virgin olive oil
  3 tablespoons red wine vinegar
  2 teaspoons dried oregano
    Salt and pepper

Cook the orzo according to package directions. Drain. Rinse under cold water and drain again. Turn the orzo into a bowl. Add the bell peppers, garlic, spinach, red onion, tomato, olives, and capers. Toss well to mix, using two spoons. Drizzle the olive oil evenly over the salad. Toss well to coat the pasta and vegetables. Drizzle the vinegar evenly over the salad. Toss well to mix. Sprinkle the oregano over the salad and salt and pepper to taste. Toss well to mix. Taste for seasonings. Serve immediately or chilled. Toss again before serving.

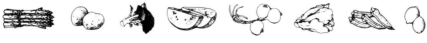

Spanish Pasta Salad with White Beans and Vegetables

SERVES 6

*At **Claire's**, we participate in an international exchange program that gives us the opportunity to employ foreign students each summer. One year we had the pleasure of employing Alberto Lopez, who is from Madrid. He brought with him a strong work ethic, a great sense of humor, and a real love for good, homemade food. This recipe, which includes a classic Spanish vinegar made from sherry, is his creation.*

- 1 pound medium pasta shells
- ½ pound (1 cup) cooked or canned white kidney beans (cannellini) or great northern beans
- ¼ cup olive oil
- 4 large cloves garlic, minced
- 1 large red onion (Bermuda), finely chopped
- 3 large red bell peppers, seeded and cut into ½-inch pieces
- 3 large ripe tomatoes, cut into ½-inch cubes
- 3 tablespoons sherry wine vinegar
- Salt and pepper

Cook the pasta shells according to package directions. Drain, rinse under cold water, and drain again. Turn into a large bowl. Add the white beans. Heat the olive oil in a large skillet over medium heat. Add the garlic, onion, and bell peppers. Cover and cook for about 5 minutes, stirring occasionally until the peppers are crisp-tender. Add the tomatoes, vinegar, and salt and pepper to taste. Stir to mix. Add the vegetables to the pasta and beans. Toss gently but thoroughly to mix well, using two spoons. Taste for seasonings. Serve immediately or chilled.

Pasta Salad Copenhagen

SERVES 8

One of the many joys of running a restaurant across from a world-class institution like Yale University is getting to meet people from all over the world. And if, like me, you are lucky enough to employ some of these people, then you can learn about the foods they eat. Kirsten Kvist Hansen worked at **Claire's Corner Copia** *for two years. She always claimed that a Danish touch could benefit most dishes, and she proved it many times over as she cooked one delicious dish after another. This salad uses traditional Danish ingredients: Havarti cheese, cucumbers, onions, and dill. The mustard-lemon dressing enhances the flavors.*

 1 pound small pasta shells
 1 large English (seedless) cucumber, cut into ½-inch cubes
 2 small onions, sliced into thin rings and separated
 1 large tomato, diced, juices included
 8 ounces dill Havarti cheese, cut into ¼-inch cubes
 1 tablespoon extra-virgin olive oil

Dressing:

 2 tablespoons spicy brown mustard
 2 lemons, squeezed, about ¼ cup juice
1¼ cups fat-free sour cream
 3 tablespoons chopped fresh dill *or* 1 tablespoon dried dillweed
    Salt and pepper

Cook the pasta according to package directions. Drain. Run under cold water, then drain again. Meanwhile, place the cucumber, onions, tomato, and Havarti in a large bowl. Add the cooked pasta. Add the oil. Toss well with two spoons to mix the ingredients and to distribute the oil evenly.

Prepare the dressing: In a medium bowl combine the mustard, lemon juice, sour cream, dill, and salt and pepper to taste. Whisk together until blended. Taste for seasonings. Add the dressing to the pasta salad. Toss well to combine. Taste for seasonings. Serve immediately or chilled. Toss again just before serving.

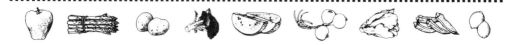

Pasta Salad with Asparagus and Pecans in a Citrus Vinaigrette

SERVES 8

Asparagus and pecans are delicious together, and when you combine them with tiny cubes of firm tofu gently tossed in an orange- and lime-flavored vinaigrette you have a healthful and beautiful dish.

1 pound medium pasta shells
2 pounds thin asparagus, tough bottoms removed, cut in 1-inch pieces
1 pound firm tofu, drained and cut into ¼-inch cubes
1 large ripe tomato, diced
¼ cup pecan halves
3 tablespoons extra-virgin olive oil
½ large orange, squeezed, about ½ cup juice
1 tablespoon grated lime zest
2 limes, squeezed, about 3 tablespoons juice
1 large shallot, minced
¼ cup soy milk
  Salt and pepper

Bring 6 quarts of lightly salted water to a boil in a large covered pot over high heat. Stir in the pasta shells. After the pasta has cooked to within 5 minutes of the cooking time according to the package directions, add the asparagus. Continue cooking for 5 minutes, stirring occasionally, until the pasta is cooked and the asparagus is crisp-tender. Drain the pasta and asparagus. Rinse under cold water then drain again. Turn into a bowl. Add the tofu, tomato, and pecans. Toss gently but thoroughly to combine, using two spoons.

In a separate bowl, whisk together the olive oil, orange juice, lime zest, lime juice, and shallot. Slowly add the soy milk, whisking to combine. Whisk in salt and pepper to taste. Pour this over the pasta salad. Toss well to coat, using two spoons. Taste for seasonings. Serve immediately or chilled.

    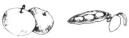

Pasta Salad with Artichoke Hearts, Green Peas, and Hearts of Palm in a Creamy Garlic and Basil Dressing

SERVES 8

This delicious pasta salad is my choice for those nights when I want a quick and easy dish for dinner. Add a simple tossed salad and some good bread and you're all set.

- 1 pound medium pasta shells
- 1 teaspoon olive oil
- 1 10-ounce package frozen petite green peas, defrosted
- 1 14-ounce can artichoke hearts, drained and quartered
- 7 ounces canned hearts of palm, drained and cut into ¼-inch slices

Dressing:

- 1 cup soy milk
- 2 large cloves garlic, chopped
- 1 cup packed fresh basil leaves
- ½ cup dairy-free or low-fat mayonnaise (you can find soy mayonnaise at health food stores)
  Salt and pepper
- ¼ cup chopped pecans

Cook the pasta shells according to package directions. Drain, rinse under cold water, then drain again. Turn into a large bowl. Drizzle the olive oil over the pasta. Toss well to prevent the pasta from sticking. Add the peas, artichoke hearts, and hearts of palm. Toss well to mix. Set aside while you prepare the dressing. Place the soy milk, garlic, and basil leaves in a blender. Cover. Blend on high speed for 15 seconds to combine. Add the mayonnaise, and salt and pepper to taste. Cover and pulse 10 times to blend. Taste for seasonings. Pour the dressing over the pasta salad. Toss well using two spoons. Add the pecans. Toss again to mix. Taste for seasonings.

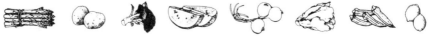

Waldorf Pasta Salad
SERVES 8

*I was thrilled when our general manager, Chrissy, made a Waldorf salad one summer day at **Claire's**. I'm happy to say that this new salad is delicious, cholesterol-free, and (if you use the new non-dairy sour cream available in health food stores) it can also be lactose-free. If you have never eaten jicama, ask for it in your produce section. It should be available year-round. It is a root vegetable with a thin pale brown skin and crunchy flesh. Peel it with a paring knife.*

   1 pound medium pasta shells
   1 medium jicama (about 2¼ pounds), peeled and cut into ½-inch cubes
   4 ribs celery, cut into ¼-inch slices
   1 Granny Smith apple, cored, peeled, and cut into ½-inch cubes
   1 medium red apple, peeled, cored, and cut into ½-inch cubes
   2 cups seedless green grapes
   ½ cup golden raisins
   ½ cup pecan halves
   1 medium carrot, peeled and finely chopped

Dressing:

   ½ cup non-dairy mayonnaise (I use Nayonaise brand, found in health food stores) or cholesterol-free mayonnaise
   1 cup soy milk (found in health food stores and most supermarkets)
   ½ cup fat-free sour cream or yogurt
   ⅛ teaspoon ground nutmeg
   1 teaspoon ground cinnamon
   ⅛ teaspoon ground ginger
   1 tablespoon firmly packed dark brown sugar
      Salt and pepper

Cook the pasta shells according to the package directions. Drain well, then rinse under cold water. Drain again, then turn into a large bowl. Add the jicama, celery, apple, grapes, raisins, pecans, and carrot. Toss gently to mix with two spoons. Set aside while you prepare the dressing. In a bowl, combine the dressing ingredients. Whisk well to mix. Pour over the salad. Toss well to mix. Taste for seasonings.

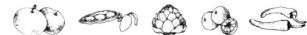

Summer Pasta Salad with Ricotta Cheese, Tomatoes, and Basil

SERVES 6

Ricotta salata is a sheep's milk cheese firm enough to cut into cubes or grate. My grandmother used to cut this cheese into tiny cubes and toss it with beautiful, fragrant summer tomatoes and basil fresh from my grandfather's garden. This makes a splendid summer lunch or a light supper at an outdoor concert.

  1 pound penne pasta
  6 to 8 ounces ricotta salata, cut into tiny cubes
  3 large ripe tomatoes, cut into ½-inch cubes
10 to 12 large fresh basil leaves
  ¼ cup extra-virgin olive oil
    Salt and pepper

Cook the pasta according to package directions. Drain. Rinse under cold water. Drain again. Turn into a bowl. Add the ricotta salata, tomatoes, and basil. Toss gently, but thoroughly, using two spoons. Drizzle the olive oil over the salad. Toss gently but thoroughly to coat evenly. Stir in salt and pepper to taste. Serve immediately or chilled.

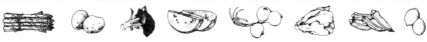

Fresh Tomato Salad

SERVES 6

My neighbor Tina was born in Sicily and she always brings me wonderful treats from her relatives, like home-cured capers and sun-dried tomatoes. She often prepares this lovely salad for me when I visit.

    2 large ripe tomatoes, cut into ¼-inch slices
    1 tablespoon extra-virgin olive oil
    2 medium cloves garlic, minced
    1 tablespoon tiny capers, drained
    ½ teaspoon dried oregano
      Salt and pepper

Arrange the tomato slices on a platter, overlapping the slices. Drizzle the olive oil evenly over the tomatoes. Scatter the garlic, capers, and oregano evenly over the tomatoes. Sprinkle lightly with salt and generously with pepper. Serve immediately or chilled.

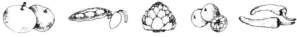

Whole-Meal Salad with Granny Smith Apples and Tofu Hot Dogs in a Creamy Curry and Lime Dressing

SERVES 4

This delicious and substantial salad is tossed in a luscious dressing made with dairy-free mayonnaise, fresh lime juice, minced shallots, and a little curry powder. You will love this delicately flavored, cholesterol-free meal in a bowl.

- ¼ pound mesclun greens or mixed baby lettuces, or 1 small head romaine, leaves torn
- 1 small endive, cut into ½-inch pieces
- ½ large English (seedless) cucumber, quartered lengthwise, then sliced into ¼-inch pieces (about 1¼ cups)
- 4 tofu hot dogs, cooked in boiling water for 1 minute, then cut into ¼-inch slices
- ¼ cup currants or golden raisins
- 1 large Granny Smith apple, cored and diced

Dressing:

- 1 cup dairy-free or soy mayonnaise (found in health food stores)
- 1 large shallot, minced
- 3 large limes, squeezed, about 4 tablespoons juice
- 1 teaspoon curry powder
- 1 teaspoon finely grated orange zest
- Salt and pepper

Combine the salad ingredients in a large bowl. Toss well to mix, using two spoons. Prepare the dressing: In a medium bowl, combine the mayonnaise, shallot, lime juice, curry powder, and orange zest. Add salt and pepper to taste. Whisk together to mix ingredients. Pour the dressing over the salad, using a rubber spatula to scrape the dressing from the bowl. Toss the salad and dressing together to coat evenly. Serve immediately, leave at room temperature, or refrigerate for up to 2 hours, then toss again before serving.

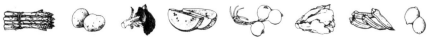

Russian Salad from Minsk

SERVES 6

This is another simple, delicious Russian salad from Natasha, who has recently immigrated to south Florida from Minsk. The combination of brine, crunch, and cream is marvelous.

- 3 medium tomatoes, cut into ½-inch cubes (juices included)
- 2 medium cucumbers, peeled, seeded, and cut into ¼-inch slices
- 6 dill gherkin pickles, chopped
- 1½ cups frozen green peas, defrosted
- ½ cup low-fat sour cream
  Salt and pepper

Combine the tomatoes and their juices, the cucumbers, pickles, and peas in a bowl. Toss gently to mix. Add the sour cream. Toss gently but thoroughly to combine. Stir in salt and pepper to taste. Serve immediately or chilled.

Balsamic Vinaigrette

MAKES ABOUT 3¼ CUPS

Balsamic vinegar is Italy's premier vinegar, made from white Trebbiano grapes and aged in barrels made from different types of woods like juniper, cherry, oak, and chestnut. I always have this delicious, simple dressing on hand. It's terrific on a tossed salad, or as a dressing for a pasta salad, and it is perfect for basting roasted or grilled eggplant, potatoes, or veggie burgers. My mom uses this dressing to marinate her chicken and to baste her fish.

2 cups extra-virgin olive oil
1 cup balsamic vinegar
¼ cup sweet vermouth
1 large shallot, minced
   Salt and pepper

Combine the ingredients in a bowl. Whisk well to mix. Taste for seasonings. Cover and refrigerate for up to one month. Shake well before using.

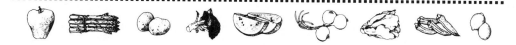

Whole-Meal Potato Salad

SERVES 6

This delicious combination makes a perfect lunch or light dinner. It travels well, which makes it a perfect picnic meal, too. Tempeh has a robust, nutty flavor. It is rich in valuable soy protein.

6 large potatoes
2 teaspoons peanut oil
1 8-ounce package tempeh, cut into ¼-inch cubes (found in health food stores)
1 medium red (Bermuda) onion, finely chopped
2 cups frozen tiny peas, defrosted
1 small cucumber, peeled, halved, seeded, and cut into ¼-inch slices
1 cup soy milk
1 large shallot, minced
2 tablespoons cider vinegar
1 tablespoon curry powder
¼ teaspoon ground red pepper (cayenne)
1 cup dairy-free or soy mayonnaise (found in health food stores)
Salt and pepper

Cook the unpeeled potatoes in an uncovered pot of lightly salted boiling water until just fork-tender, about 35 minutes. Drain and set aside until cool enough to handle. Then peel off the skins with your fingers; they should slip off easily. Cut the potatoes into quarters lengthwise, then into ¼-inch slices. Turn the potatoes into a large bowl.

Heat the peanut oil in a large skillet over medium heat. Add the tempeh and cook each side about 5 to 7 minutes until golden brown, turning to evenly brown all sides. Add the browned tempeh to the potatoes and toss gently with two spoons. Add the onion, green peas, and cucumber. Toss gently to mix.

Put the soy milk, shallot, cider vinegar, curry powder, cayenne, and mayonnaise into a mixing bowl; add salt and pepper to taste. Whisk well to combine. Taste for seasonings. Pour dressing over the potato salad, using a rubber spatula to scrape the bowl. Toss the salad and dressing to coat evenly, using two spoons.

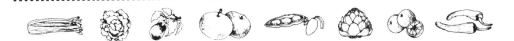

Pennsylvania Dutch Potato Salad

SERVES 8

When my friend Audrey Boyce gave me a classic German-style potato salad recipe from a Pennsylvania Dutch friend of hers, I was eager to make a vegetarian version. Fakin' Bacon is the meatless bacon I use for this recipe (you can buy it at a health food store and keep a supply on hand in your freezer); the flavor is rich and meaty without any cholesterol.

8 medium potatoes
2 tablespoons soybean margarine (found in health food stores) or canola oil
2 tablespoons olive oil
1 6-ounce package Fakin' Bacon or other meatless bacon, cut into 1-inch pieces
4 ribs celery, minced
4 medium onions, sliced into thin rings
½ cup white vinegar
¼ cup sugar
   Salt and pepper

Cook the unpeeled potatoes in an uncovered pot of lightly salted boiling water for about 40 minutes, until fork-tender. Drain and set aside. When the potatoes are cool enough to handle, peel off the skin (it should slip off easily), using your fingers. Cut the potatoes into ½-inch slices. Arrange the slices of potatoes in a large bowl, overlapping slightly.

Heat the margarine and olive oil in a 5-quart pot over low-medium heat. Add the meatless bacon, celery, and onions. Cover and cook slowly, stirring occasionally, for 20 minutes until the onions and celery are soft. Add the vinegar and sugar. Remove from the heat and stir until the sugar is dissolved. Pour dressing over the potatoes. Add salt and pepper to taste. Toss the potatoes gently but thoroughly to coat evenly, using two spoons. Taste for seasonings. Serve warm.

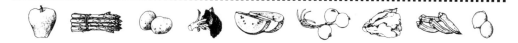

Russian Potato Salad

SERVES 8 AS AN ENTREE

Talking to new people about food is my favorite way to learn about recipes. In fact, as I was having a manicure one day, the young manicurist told me that she was from Minsk, Russia. In her rich and beautiful accent, she asked what I did for a living. She recoiled when I told her that I cooked, saying "I hate to cook." So I asked her if she liked to eat. "I love to eat . . . but I hate to cook" was her response. Before long, she was telling me all about her favorite salad that her mother makes. This salad has become wildly popular both in my restaurant and in my home.

8 medium potatoes
2 medium carrots, finely diced
4 meatless hot dogs
2 hard-cooked eggs, chopped
1 medium onion, finely chopped
8 dill gherkin pickles, cut in ¼-inch slices
1 cup dairy-free or fat-free mayonnaise (found in health food stores)
   Salt and pepper

Bring a covered pot of lightly salted water to a boil. Carefully add the unpeeled potatoes to the boiling water. Cook, uncovered, for about 30 minutes, until fork-tender. Drain the potatoes, and when cool enough to handle, remove the skin. The skin should peel off easily with your fingers. Cut the potatoes in quarters lengthwise, then cut into ¾-inch slices. Place in a large bowl.

While the potatoes are cooking, bring a small pot of water to a boil. Add the diced carrots, cover, and cook for about 2 minutes until just tender. Add the hot dogs. Cover and remove the pan from the heat. Set aside for 2 minutes, then drain. Remove the hot dogs and cut into ¼-inch slices. Add the sliced hot dogs and the cooked carrots to the potatoes. Add the hard-cooked eggs, onion, and pickles. Toss gently but thoroughly to mix, using two spoons. Add the mayonnaise. Toss gently but thoroughly to mix. Mix in the salt and pepper to taste. Serve immediately or chilled.

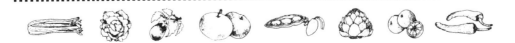

Sweet Potato Salad

SERVES 6

This salad is a nice change from potato salads made with white potatoes, and it goes just as well with a savory veggie burger.

- 4 large sweet potatoes, peeled and cut into medium chunks
- 1 small sweet onion, cut into thin rings and separated
- ⅓ cup dried cranberries or cherries (found in most supermarkets, gourmet stores, and health food stores)
- 2 tablespoons extra-virgin olive oil
- 1 tablespoon apple cider vinegar
- 1 lime, squeezed, about 2 tablespoons juice
- ¼ teaspoon allspice
- ⅛ teaspoon ground red pepper (cayenne)
- ¼ teaspoon dried thyme
- Salt and pepper

Cook the sweet potatoes in lightly salted boiling water, for about 10 minutes or until fork-tender. Drain well. Turn into a bowl. Add the onion and dried cranberries. Toss gently to mix. Into a separate bowl, add the olive oil, cider vinegar, lime juice, allspice, cayenne, and thyme. Whisk together until well blended. Whisk in salt and pepper to taste. Pour the dressing evenly over the potatoes. Toss gently but thoroughly to evenly coat the potatoes with the dressing. Taste for seasonings. Serve immediately or chilled.

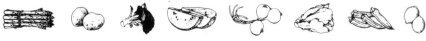

Italian Green Bean and Potato Salad

SERVES 8 (OR MORE)

My mom has made this traditional Italian-style potato salad for as long as I can remember. In fact, I can't remember a picnic without it. And now that green beans are available year-round, you can enjoy this salad often. Serve it warm as a side dish with dinner. Warm or cold, it's delicious!

6 medium potatoes, peeled and cut into 1-inch chunks
1 pound green beans, trimmed and cut into 2-inch pieces
1 large red (Bermuda) onion, cut in half lengthwise, then into thin slices
¼ cup extra-virgin olive oil
5 tablespoons red wine vinegar
2 teaspoons dried oregano
   Salt and pepper

Cook the potatoes and the green beans together in lightly salted boiling water for about 15 minutes, until the potatoes are fork-tender. Drain well. Turn the potatoes and green beans into a large bowl. Set aside for about 15 minutes to cool down slightly. Add the onion and toss well with two spoons. Drizzle the olive oil evenly over the top and toss well.

Drizzle the vinegar over the salad and toss well. Sprinkle the oregano, salt, and pepper evenly over the salad. Toss well to combine. Taste for seasonings. Serve at room temperature or chilled. Toss again right before serving.

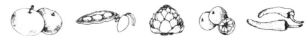

French Potato Salad

SERVES 6

*My dear friend Joan Brett owns and operates the Cooking School of the Rockies, where I had the distinct pleasure of teaching my first cooking class ever. The experience was magical! Of course, the magnificent view of the foothills of the Rockies didn't hurt any, but I also learned a great deal from Joan about teaching and sharing information. We spent three days together talking and eating. She told me about her French potato salad, which reminded me of the one I used to prepare at **Claire's** when we first opened in 1975. The dry vermouth in the dressing gives this salad its great flavor.*

> 6 medium potatoes
> 1 large sweet onion (preferably Vidalia), sliced into thin rings
> 1 large shallot, minced
> ¼ cup chopped fresh Italian flat-leaf parsley

Dressing:

> 3 tablespoons olive oil
> 2 limes, squeezed, about 3 tablespoons juice
> 1 tablespoon Dijon mustard
> 3 tablespoons dry vermouth
> 2 tablespoons chopped fresh thyme *or* 2 teaspoons dried
> Salt and pepper

Cook the unpeeled potatoes in an uncovered pot of lightly salted boiling water for about 30 minutes or until fork-tender. Drain and set aside until they cool down enough to handle comfortably. Remove the skin from the potatoes with your fingers; it should pull off easily. Cut the potatoes into ½-inch slices. Place them in a large mixing bowl. Add the onion rings, shallot, and parsley. Gently toss to mix using two spoons. In a separate bowl combine the olive oil, lime juice, mustard, vermouth, thyme, and salt and pepper to taste. Whisk together to mix thoroughly. Taste for seasonings. Pour the dressing over the potatoes. Gently toss until the salad is evenly coated with the dressing. Taste for seasonings. Serve immediately or chilled. Toss again just before serving.

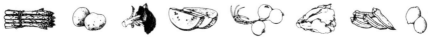

Creamy Tofu Salad with Grapes, Jicama, and Pecans

SERVES 4 TO 8

This salad has a touch of curry and lime juice in the dressing, which goes nicely with the sweet and crunchy ingredients. You can serve it as a salad or a sandwich filling—it's wonderful on raisin bread. Jicama ("hick-a-ma") is a Mexican tuber rich in vitamin C, with a pleasant crunchy texture and a taste like Granny Smith apples and water chestnuts combined. You can find jicama in the produce section of most supermarkets.

1 pound firm tofu, drained, cut into ½-inch cubes
1 cup seedless green grapes, cut in half lengthwise
¼ medium jicama, peeled and cut into ½-inch cubes
1 Granny Smith apple, cored and cut into ½-inch cubes
½ cup pecan halves
1 small sweet onion, finely chopped

Dressing:

½ cup dairy-free or soy mayonnaise (found in health food stores)
2 tablespoons soy milk
2 large limes, squeezed, about 3 tablespoons juice
2 teaspoons curry powder
2 tablespoons Major Grey's mango chutney
Salt and pepper

Place the tofu, grapes, jicama, apple, pecans, and onion in a large bowl. Toss gently to mix, using two spoons. In a separate bowl, whisk together the mayonnaise, soy milk, lime juice, curry powder, and chutney until smooth. Stir in salt and pepper to taste. Pour the dressing over the salad and toss well to coat evenly. Taste for seasonings. Serve immediately or chilled.

Dairy-Free Green Goddess Dressing

MAKES ABOUT 3 CUPS

During the sixties, my brother Billy worked at The Beefsteak Tavern in Branford, Connecticut. They were widely known for their mammoth prime ribs and the creamy, rich green goddess dressing that they lavished upon huge bowls full of salad. That dressing haunted me for years after they closed. I experimented with different combinations, trying to duplicate the rich flavor that I loved, only with less fat and cholesterol. I sometimes make a salad of romaine leaves and add tiny cubes of fat-free cheese, "ham," and "turkey" deli slices (tasty meatless versions, found at health food stores). I add this wonderful dressing and voila!

  1 cup soy milk
  3 large cloves garlic, minced
  ½ cup finely chopped fresh Italian flat-leaf parsley
  ¼ cup white vinegar
  ½ lemon, squeezed, about 2 tablespoons juice
  3 tablespoons finely chopped fresh chives
  1 tablespoon dried tarragon
  1 cup dairy-free or soy mayonnaise (found in health food stores)
    Salt and pepper

Put the soy milk, garlic, parsley, vinegar, lemon juice, chives, and tarragon into a blender. Cover and blend at high speed for 15 seconds, until blended, stopping once to scrape down the sides using a rubber spatula. Pour into a bowl. Whisk in the mayonnaise until smooth. Whisk in salt and pepper to taste. Cover and refrigerate.

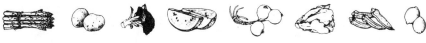

Dairy-Free Caesar Salad Dressing

MAKES ABOUT 1¾ CUPS

If you know someone who avoids dairy, make this dressing for them—they'll love you for it. Toss it with romaine leaves for a delightful salad. Many health food stores carry a delicious new dairy-free Parmesan cheese substitute that you can sprinkle on top for an added treat. At **Claire's,** *we sometimes sprinkle our Caesar salads with minced sun-dried tomatoes.*

  1 cup soy milk
  ½ cup dairy-free mayonnaise (I use Nayonaise, found in health food stores)
  5 large cloves garlic, quartered
  1 lemon, squeezed, about 3 tablespoons juice
  1 tablespoon Dijon mustard
  ½ teaspoon blackstrap molasses
  1 teaspoon cider vinegar
    Salt and pepper

Place the ingredients in a blender. Cover. Blend on high speed for 20 seconds, stopping once to scrape down the sides, using a rubber spatula. Taste for seasonings.

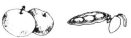

3
Appetizers and Side Dishes

- Roasted Garlic with Gorgonzola and Crostini
- Lemon-Parmesan Artichoke Hearts
- Cauliflower Pancakes
- Broiled Marinated Eggplant Rounds
- Pickled Eggplant
- Coconut Fried Oyster Mushrooms with a Mango-Lime Dipping Sauce
- Roasted Bell Peppers with Capers, Olives, and Oregano
- Southern-Style Green Beans
- Little Garlic Toasts
- Spinach and Goat Cheese Quesadillas
- Tomato Bruschetta
- Asparagus with Warm Mustard Vinaigrette
- Sautéed Green Beans, Carrots, and Shiitake Mushrooms
- Sautéed Bok Choy
- Broccoli with Garlic Chips
- Brussels Sprouts in Lemon Vinaigrette
- Sweet and Sour Red Cabbage
- German-Style Red Cabbage and Apples
- Savoy Cabbage Sautéed with Fresh Garlic
- Orange-Maple Carrots
- Roasted Carrots with Dill
- Sweet Cinnamon Carrots
- Italian-Style Sautéed Cauliflower
- Parsleyed Cauliflower

      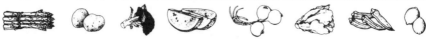

- Escarole Sautéed in Olive Oil with Garlic and Torn Bread
- Corn with Lemon, Orange, and Thyme
- Stir-Fried Asian Vegetables
- Maple-Glazed, Apple-Stuffed Acorn Squash
- Kale with Golden Raisins and Toasted Walnuts
- Portobello Mushrooms Sautéed with Olive Oil and Vermouth
- Onions Roasted with Herbs
- Gorgonzola-Stuffed Roasted Onions
- Mashed Parsnips, Sweet and White Potatoes
- Garlic Mashed Potatoes
- Scalloped Potatoes
- Mashed Sweet Potatoes
- Candied Sweet Potatoes
- Sautéed Spinach with Golden Raisins and Toasted Pine Nuts
- Spinach and Leeks in Pernod
- Roasted Fennel and Tomatoes
- Herbed Barley with Almonds
- Sautéed Zucchini Spears
- Refried Black Beans
- White Beans Stewed with Tomatoes and Sage
- Fresh Corn Polenta with Tomatoes and Basil Ricotta
- Fresh Corn-Cilantro Cornbread
- Kasha with Sautéed Mushrooms and Onions
- Matzo Brei
- Basmati Rice with Green Peas and Pine Nuts
- Basmati Rice Pilaf
- Leban (Lebanese Yogurt)
- Tequila-Lime Sauce
- Portobello and Cremini Mushroom and Herb Gravy
- Cranberry-Lime Sauce
- Sawmill Gravy
- Biscuits

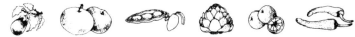

Roasted Garlic with Gorgonzola and Crostini

SERVES 8

Roasted garlic has many marvelous uses. At home I serve it along with slices of toasted bread (crostini) and good cheese for a lovely appetizer. I also use roasted garlic as a spread on sliced bread, with slices of native tomatoes, olive oil, and basil leaves, for a delicious sandwich. Roasted garlic has a wonderful, mellow flavor, and I often find that even those people who avoid garlic as a rule will eat and enjoy this more delicate approach to garlic.

I highly recommend clay garlic roasters for their convenience and they do look attractive centered on a plate, surrounded by toasted bread and cheese. You can, however, use tin foil to enclose your garlic for roasting.

- 2 large bulbs garlic
- 2 teaspoons extra-virgin olive oil
- ¼ to ½ teaspoon dried rosemary leaves *or* 1 teaspoon fresh leaves, finely chopped
  Salt and pepper
- 1 loaf French or Italian bread, cut into ¾-inch slices, lightly toasted
- ¼ pound Gorgonzola cheese

Preheat oven to 350 degrees. On a cutting board, lay the garlic bulb on its side. Carefully cut off the tips of each clove, about ⅛ inch from top, exposing as many cloves as possible. Repeat with the other bulb of garlic. Measure 1 tablespoon of water onto the bottom dish of the roaster then arrange the bulbs of garlic in the center, not touching. Drizzle the olive oil evenly over the bulb, sprinkle the rosemary leaves, scattering them evenly, then sprinkle lightly with the salt. Grind the pepper over the top. Cover the roaster and bake for 1 hour. The garlic will be soft. Carefully set the roaster onto an oven-proof plate. Surround the garlic with the toasted bread and a wedge of Gorgonzola cheese. Remove the cover from the garlic roaster. Advise your guests to pick out and spread a clove (it should come out of its paper sack easily, using a small spreader) onto a slice of toasted bread and then top it with a piece of cheese. Enjoy it!

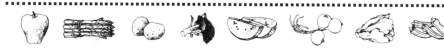

Lemon-Parmesan Artichoke Hearts

SERVES 6

These make a lovely, crisp addition to an antipasto platter or a terrific snack or appetizer with a squeeze of lemon on top. A huge serving platter of penne pasta in garlic and fresh basil-scented Marinara Sauce (page 178), encircled by these lemony, lightly fried artichoke hearts, makes a great dinner. I also love to include these little gems on a picnic because they are delicious at room temperature.

    1 14-ounce can (not marinated) artichoke hearts (about 8 hearts), drained
       and cut in half lengthwise
    ½ cup flour
       Salt and pepper
    5 eggs or equivalent egg substitute
    2 tablespoons chopped fresh Italian flat-leaf parsley
    2 cups plain dry bread crumbs
    ¼ cup olive oil
    1 lemon, squeezed, about 2 tablespoons juice
    1 tablespoon grated lemon zest
    2 tablespoons grated Parmesan cheese, or soy Parmesan (found in most
       health food stores)

Place the artichokes in a bowl. Measure the flour in another bowl. Whisk a little salt and pepper into the flour. Break the eggs into another bowl. Sprinkle with salt and pepper. Add the parsley. Beat the eggs lightly with a whisk or a fork until blended. Measure the bread crumbs into another bowl. Have a nonstick cookie sheet or a cookie sheet that has been sprayed with cooking oil spray near the stove. You'll use this for the fried artichoke hearts. Line up your bowls of flour, eggs, and bread crumbs in a row. Place a large plate next to the bread crumbs.

Using two forks, tongs, or your hands, gently roll an artichoke heart in the flour and gently shake off the excess. Roll the coated artichoke heart in the beaten eggs and carefully shake off the excess. Roll the coated artichoke heart in the bread crumbs, coating completely. Shake off the excess. Roll the coated artichoke

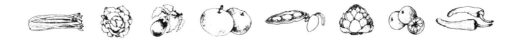

heart in the egg again, shaking off the excess, then roll it again in the bread crumbs to coat completely. Shake off the excess. Place the "double dipped" artichoke heart onto the large plate. Repeat the process with the remaining artichoke hearts.

Preheat the oven to 350 degrees. Heat the oil in a large (12-inch) nonstick skillet over medium-high heat. Arrange the breaded artichoke hearts in a single layer in the hot oil, without crowding (don't let them touch). Work in batches if necessary. Cook each side for 1 to 2 minutes, turning with tongs, until evenly browned and crisp. Transfer the cooked artichokes to the cookie sheet. After you have finished browning the artichokes, drizzle them evenly with the lemon juice. Sprinkle the lemon zest and the Parmesan cheese evenly over the top. Bake for 15 minutes, until brown and crisp.

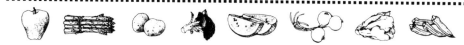

Cauliflower Pancakes

SERVES 6

I still get excited when I visit my mother and see a plateful of these beautiful cauliflower pancakes waiting on the stove. They are perfect for a picnic because they are scrumptious warm or chilled. Enjoy these delicate pancakes plain, with applesauce, or with Marinara Sauce (page 178).

   1 large cauliflower
   6 eggs or equivalent egg substitute
   ¼ cup finely chopped fresh Italian flat-leaf parsley
   ½ small onion, minced
   ¼ cup unbleached white flour
   1 teaspoon baking powder
   2 tablespoons grated Parmesan cheese
     Salt and pepper
   2 to 3 tablespoons olive oil

Remove and discard any leaves from the cauliflower. Cook the head of cauliflower in lightly salted boiling water for about 25 minutes or until soft-tender when pierced with a fork. Drain in a colander. Set aside until cool enough to handle (about 15 minutes). Cut out and discard the core of the cauliflower. Place the florets in a large bowl. Mash lightly with a potato masher, until the cauliflower is broken into tiny pieces. Add the eggs, parsley, onion, flour, baking powder, cheese, and salt and pepper to taste. Mix together with a wooden spoon, beating lightly to combine.

Heat a large nonstick skillet over low heat. Brush the skillet with about 1 teaspoon of the olive oil. Use a ¼-cup measure to scoop the pancake batter into the skillet, and flatten each pancake slightly using the back of the measuring cup. You should be able to fit 3 to 4 pancakes in the skillet without crowding. Cook the pancakes for 4 minutes without disturbing then carefully lift up the edge with a plastic spatula to check them. They are ready to turn over when the underside is a medium brown color. Carefully turn the pancakes over using two plastic spatulas. Cook the other side for 4 to 5 minutes until nicely browned. Carefully transfer the pancakes to a platter. Stir the batter in between cooking batches of the pancakes, repeating the process until all of the batter is used.

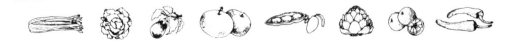

Broiled Marinated Eggplant Rounds

SERVES 6

Plates of these marvelous eggplant rounds disappear quickly in my house. We enjoy them as appetizers or as part of an antipasto platter with Pickled Eggplant (page 74) and Roasted Bell Peppers with Capers, Olives, and Oregano (page 78). They are also delicious in a sandwich with a slice of Asiago cheese. Regular purple eggplants are fine, but do try to find those beautiful, white eggplants. Their flesh is creamy smooth and they usually have fewer seeds, so you get more "meat."

    4 medium unpeeled eggplants, stems cut off
    4 tablespoons extra-virgin olive oil
    2 tablespoons balsamic vinegar
    2 large cloves garlic, minced
      Salt and pepper

Preheat the broiler. Adjust the broiler rack to the highest position. Cut eggplants into 1-inch rounds. Arrange the rounds in a single layer on a nonstick cookie sheet or on a cookie sheet sprayed with nonstick cooking oil. In a small bowl combine the olive oil, balsamic vinegar, garlic, and salt and pepper to taste. Whisk to mix. Brush about half of this mixture over the eggplant rounds with a pastry brush. Broil for about 7 minutes, until browned but not burned. Turn the eggplant rounds over to broil the other side for 4 to 5 minutes until browned and tender when pierced with a fork. Transfer to a platter, overlapping slightly. Brush the remaining marinade over the eggplant rounds. Taste for seasonings.

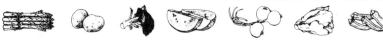

Pickled Eggplant

MAKES SIX 8-OUNCE JARS

Jars of homemade Italian pickled eggplant are great to have around. It is just so versatile. You can enjoy a forkful on top of toasted bread with a glass of wine. Pickled eggplant makes a perfect sandwich filling either alone or with roasted red peppers and sliced Fontina or provolone cheese. It makes a fine addition to your antipasto platter, along with good olives, caponata, marinated mushrooms, and artichoke hearts. And your friends and family will love you for sending them a jar, because homemade pickled eggplant is far more delicious than any commercial variety. My mother-in-law's neighbor Minnie taught me how to make this wonderful recipe and I've been making (and sharing) it several times a year. You'll need six 8-ounce jars with tight-fitting lids. I buy attractive jars for gift giving.

½ gallon white vinegar (buy a 1-gallon plastic container)
4 medium eggplants (about 4½ pounds)
   Salt
½ cup extra-virgin olive oil
1 large bulb garlic (10 to 12 cloves), coarsely chopped
2 tablespoons drained hot cherry peppers in oil, chopped
½ teaspoon dried oregano leaves
   Freshly ground black pepper

Clean and dry your jars. Set aside. Pour the vinegar into an 8-quart pot. Cover and bring to a simmer. Lower heat and just keep warm while you proceed with the recipe. Peel the eggplants and trim the ends. Cut each eggplant in half lengthwise. Slice one half into ¼-inch slices, then stack and slice widthwise into ⅛-inch strips. As you cut each half, place in a bowl and sprinkle liberally with salt and toss well to mix. Repeat this process of slicing, salting, and tossing until all of the eggplant has been sliced. You will be adding what seems like a lot of salt, but the vinegar bath will remove any overly salty taste.

By the time you finish slicing the eggplant it will have released a lot of dark liquid. Raise the heat under your pot of vinegar so that it is simmering. You'll need to work quickly for the next 5 minutes or so. You might want to turn on your answering machine and avoid any interruptions. Remove the cover and pick up a handful of the eggplant and squeeze out as much liquid as you can, then carefully lower the eggplant into the pot of simmering vinegar. Continue squeezing out the liquid from the handfuls of eggplant and adding them to the vinegar. Stir the eggplant around briefly, using a non-aluminum slotted spoon. Immediately but carefully drain the eggplant in a non-aluminum colander set in the sink. Squeeze out as much vinegar as you can. It helps to place a plastic plate or round cover over the eggplant, then use the 1-gallon plastic vinegar container to press on the plate, squeezing out as much excess liquid as possible. Turn the eggplant into a bowl. Add the olive oil, garlic, hot cherry peppers, oregano, and pepper to taste. Toss well to combine. Taste for seasonings. Pack the eggplant into the 6 jars, leaving 1 inch of space on the top. Cover and lightly tighten the lids. Set aside in a cool, dry place (unrefrigerated) for 5 days. The eggplant will absorb some of the olive oil, so each day add enough olive oil to cover the eggplant. Cover tightly and label. Store in your refrigerator. Pickled Eggplant will keep well for one month to two months. Serve chilled or at room temperature.

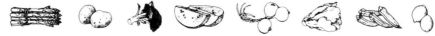

Coconut Fried Oyster Mushrooms with a Mango-Lime Dipping Sauce

SERVES 8

I feel compelled to warn you that it's not easy to stop eating these tasty little Caribbean-style treats. As soon as you dip your first mushroom into the mango-lime sauce, you'll see what I mean.

1 cup flour
¼ teaspoon ground red pepper (cayenne)
1 teaspoon ground ginger
Salt and black pepper
1½ cups unsweetened coconut milk
1½ cups plain dry bread crumbs
1½ cups unsweetened coconut
8 ounces oyster mushrooms, rinsed and patted dry
½ cup peanut oil

Mango-Lime Sauce:

1 ripe mango, peeled, pitted, and sliced
2 limes, squeezed, about 3 tablespoons
2 teaspoons balsamic vinegar
¼ teaspoon ground red pepper (cayenne)
1 tablespoon chopped fresh cilantro

Measure the flour, cayenne, and ginger into a bowl. Sprinkle with salt and black pepper. Whisk together to mix. Pour the coconut milk into a separate, shallow bowl. Measure the bread crumbs and the coconut into a third bowl and whisk together to mix. Set a nonstick cookie sheet next to the bread crumb mixture for placing the mushrooms after you've dipped them. Pick up a mushroom by the stem and dredge it in the flour. Shake off the excess. Dip the mushroom into the coconut milk, turning to coat if necessary. Shake off the excess. Dip the

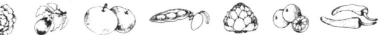

mushroom into the bread crumb mixture, turning to coat completely. Place the coated mushroom on the cookie sheet and repeat the process until all of the mushrooms are breaded.

Set a serving platter by the stove. Heat 2 tablespoons of the oil in a large non-stick skillet over medium heat. Arrange as many mushrooms as will fit in a single layer, leaving space in between. Do not crowd the mushrooms or the oil will cool down and the mushrooms will taste greasy. Cook each side for 2 to 3 minutes until brown, then turn over with a plastic spatula or tongs to brown the other side. Transfer the browned mushrooms to the platter. Carefully remove the skillet from the stove. While wearing oven mitts, wipe out the skillet with paper towels. Heat another 2 tablespoons of oil over medium heat and repeat the process of pan-frying until all of the mushrooms are cooked. Set aside while you prepare the mango-lime sauce.

Place the mango, lime juice, balsamic vinegar, cayenne, and cilantro into a blender cup. Cover and pulse on high speed about 15 times until fairly smooth, stopping once to scrape down the sides with a rubber spatula. Serve this sauce with the mushrooms for dipping.

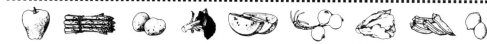

Roasted Bell Peppers with Capers, Olives, and Oregano

SERVES 6

Roasted peppers are delicious! They are also loaded with vitamin C and are rich in fiber. And as though that isn't enough to make you run right to the kitchen, there's also the fact that they are easy to prepare and versatile. Roasted peppers are delightful in a sandwich on Italian bread, they make a luscious addition to an antipasto platter, and you can slice them into thick strips and toss them with pasta, additional olive oil, and fresh garlic for a quick dinner entree.

> 4 bell peppers, mixed red, yellow, and green
> 1 tablespoon tiny capers, drained
> 12 oil-cured black olives, pitted
> 1 large clove garlic, minced
> ½ teaspoon dried oregano
> 1 tablespoon extra-virgin olive oil
>   Salt and pepper

Preheat broiler to the highest heat. Adjust broiler rack to the highest position. Rinse and drain the peppers. Cut each pepper in half lengthwise. Seed the peppers by holding a pepper half, cut-side up in one hand. With your other hand, hold your thumb over the base of the stem, reach your fingers over and around the seeds and core, and lift out the seed bundle and stem all at once. Discard the stem, seed, and core. While still holding the pepper half, tap it, cut-side down, onto the palm of your free hand, releasing the remaining seeds. With your fingers, gently tear out the soft, white ribs inside the pepper half (they taste bitter). Repeat this process with the remaining pepper halves.

Rinse and drain the peppers again. Arrange the pepper halves, cut-side down, on a nonstick sheet pan (with sides, to collect the juices) or on a sheet pan that has been coated with nonstick cooking spray. Broil with the door open about 5 inches, for about 12 minutes, rotating the pan from front to back after about 8 minutes, until the tops of the peppers are slightly shriveled and charred. Remove the pan from the broiler and, using tongs, turn each pepper half to the other side.

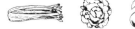   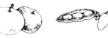

Broil the other side for about 4 to 5 minutes, until the skin is charred and the pepper is shriveled slightly.

Remove the peppers from the broiler and place the peppers and their juices in a bowl. Cover the bowl tightly with plastic wrap. Set the bowl aside for about 30 minutes, until the peppers have "steamed" and are cool enough to handle. Carefully peel off the charred skin with your fingers; it should come off easily. I leave most of the uncharred skin on, but if you prefer, peel off all of the skin, using a paring knife on the skin that does not come off easily. Arrange the pepper halves on a serving plate. Pour any juices over the top. Scatter the capers, olives, and garlic over the peppers. Sprinkle the oregano evenly over the top. Drizzle with the olive oil. Sprinkle lightly with salt and pepper to taste. Serve immediately or cover and refrigerate. They are delicious served either chilled or at room temperature.

Southern-Style Green Beans

SERVES 6

My friend Sue Penn told me about the southern-style, slow-cooked green beans she enjoyed as a child in South Carolina. Enjoy them as part of a traditional southern meal of Chicken-Fried Vegetable Burgers with Sawmill Gravy (page 183) and Biscuits (page 126).

- 4 quarts water
- 1 pound green beans, trimmed
- 3 tablespoons olive oil
- 2 medium sweet onions, finely chopped
- 1 package meatless bacon (found in health food stores), coarsely chopped
  Salt and pepper

Boil the water and cook the green beans for about 10 minutes or until crisp-tender. Drain. Heat the olive oil in a large deep skillet over medium heat. Add the onions and the meatless bacon. Cover and cook for 15 minutes, stirring occasionally, until the onions are soft. Stir in the cooked green beans, and salt and pepper to taste, mixing well to coat evenly. Cook, stirring occasionally, for 3 minutes until the green beans are tender. Taste for seasonings.

Little Garlic Toasts

MAKES ABOUT 32 TOASTS

My mom always keeps a basket of plain little toasts (crostini) in her kitchen. Sometimes she makes them for bean soups and onion soup, or tops them with vegetables or cheese for a satisfying snack any time of day. I love little garlic toasts in a bowl with White Beans Stewed with Tomatoes and Sage (page 114) on top.

1 loaf French or Italian bread, cut into ¼-inch slices
4 large cloves garlic, cut in half lengthwise
1 tablespoon extra-virgin olive oil
  Salt and pepper

Place the cooking rack on the highest shelf of the broiler. Preheat the broiler to high. *Gently* rub the cut sides of the garlic onto both sides of each slice of bread. Place on a cookie sheet. Toast under the broiler for about 1 minute until golden brown. Remove from the oven and carefully turn over each slice of bread. Return to the broiler and toast the breads about 1 minute more, until golden brown. Remove from the broiler. Brush the olive oil evenly over the top of the toasts. Sprinkle lightly with salt and pepper.

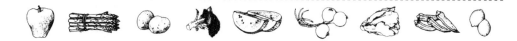

Spinach and Goat Cheese Quesadillas

SERVES 6 ENTREE SERVINGS OR 12 APPETIZERS

Quesadillas are like savory Mexican grilled cheese sandwiches—and they are so versatile. Serve them with a tossed salad with a handful of chick-peas on top for added fiber and protein, and you will have a delicious and quick weeknight supper. Or invite your friends over after work for quesadillas and a glass of wine to unwind after a busy day.

2 tablespoons plus 1 teaspoon olive oil
4 large cloves garlic, minced
1 10-ounce bag fresh spinach, well washed and chopped
   Salt and pepper
6 10-inch flour tortillas
4 ounces goat cheese, crumbled

Preheat the oven to 350 degrees. Heat 2 tablespoons of the oil in a large skillet over a low-medium heat. Add the garlic and spinach. Sprinkle with salt and pepper to taste. Cover and cook for about 5 minutes, stirring occasionally, until the spinach is cooked. Arrange 3 flour tortillas in a single layer on a nonstick cookie sheet, or spray a cookie sheet with cooking spray. Using a slotted spoon, arrange the spinach mixture evenly over the tortillas.

Scatter the goat cheese evenly over the spinach. Top each spinach quesadilla with a tortilla. Press down lightly. Brush the tops of the tortillas with the remaining 1 teaspoon of oil. Bake for about 12 minutes, until the quesadillas are barely golden brown. Cut into wedges to serve. Serve immediately.

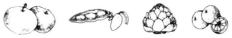

Tomato Bruschetta

SERVES 8

While growing up, I remember my mom always keeping a covered tin of lightly toasted, sliced, Italian bread rounds on hand for quick snacks. (Simply arrange slices of bread in a single layer on a cookie sheet and toast under the broiler for about 1 minute, then turn using tongs and toast the other side.) She would top them with a spoonful of ricotta or just spread them with some butter or olive oil, a slice of tomato, and a sprinkle of salt. I have carried on this tradition and during the summer I never miss an opportunity to use the magnificent summer tomatoes for my bruschetta. This dish makes a lovely appetizer, and it requires only basic staples, which makes it a perfect choice for unexpected guests. My husband likes to spread a thin layer of goat cheese or ricotta on the toasted bread before topping with the tomato mixture. It's a delicious variation you should try.

  1 large tomato, diced (about ½-inch cubes)
  ¼ small, sweet onion, finely diced (about ¼-inch pieces)
  4 to 6 fresh basil leaves, minced
  2 tablespoons minced, fresh Italian flat-leaf parsley
  1 to 2 tablespoons extra-virgin olive oil
     Salt and pepper
  1 loaf French or Italian bread, cut into ¾-inch slices, lightly toasted

Place the diced tomatoes, onion, basil, parsley, olive oil, salt, and pepper in a bowl. Toss gently to mix. Taste for seasonings. Spoon a heaping tablespoon of this mixture on top of the toasted bread slices and arrange on a serving dish. Grind a little more pepper over each bruschetta. Serve immediately.

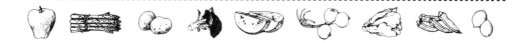

Asparagus with Warm Mustard Vinaigrette

SERVES 6

Have plenty of good bread on hand to sop up the luscious sauce in this lovely, French-inspired asparagus dish.

- ¼ cup water
- 2 pounds thin asparagus, tough bottoms removed
  Salt and pepper

Dressing:

- 2 tablespoons extra-virgin olive oil
- 1 tablespoon Dijon mustard
- 2 tablespoons sherry vinegar
- 1 large shallot, minced
  Salt and pepper

Bring the water to a boil in a large, nonstick skillet over high heat. Carefully arrange the asparagus spears in the boiling water using tongs. Sprinkle with salt and pepper. Cover and cook for 5 to 7 minutes, until the water has absorbed and the asparagus is just tender. Remove from the heat. Into a small bowl, measure the olive oil, mustard, vinegar, and salt and pepper to taste. Whisk to blend well. Pour this over the warm asparagus. Toss gently but thoroughly to coat evenly, using two spoons. Taste for seasonings. Serve warm.

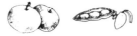

Sautéed Green Beans, Carrots, and Shiitake Mushrooms

SERVES 6

This colorful and crunchy combination of Asian ingredients and flavors is one of my favorites.

- 2 tablespoons peanut oil
- 4 large cloves garlic, thinly sliced
- 1 pound green beans, trimmed
  Salt and pepper
- 3 medium carrots, peeled and cut into matchstick pieces
- 10 medium shiitake mushrooms, stems removed and discarded, caps thinly sliced
- 1 tablespoon soy sauce

Heat the oil in a large skillet over medium heat. Add the garlic. Cook for 3 minutes, stirring frequently until softened but not brown. Add the green beans. Sprinkle with salt and pepper to taste. Cover and cook for 7 minutes, stirring occasionally, until crisp-tender. Stir in the carrots, mushrooms, and soy sauce. Cover and cook for 3 to 5 minutes, stirring occasionally, until the green beans are tender. Taste for seasonings.

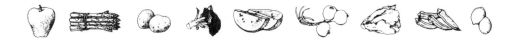

Sautéed Bok Choy

SERVES 4

Bok choy is shaped like a bunch of celery, only the stalks are thick and creamy white and the leaves are long and very dark green. Many supermarkets call bok choy "Chinese cabbage," but other stores give that name to napa cabbage, a different vegetable altogether. Don't worry about the name, just look for the beautiful dark-green bunches, and cook with them often because they are delicious and rich in vitamins C and A.

1 large bunch bok choy (about 1¾ pounds)
1 tablespoon peanut oil
3 large cloves garlic, finely chopped
¼ cup coarsely chopped almonds
1 inch fresh ginger, peeled and minced
¼ teaspoon crushed red pepper
   Salt and pepper
1 tablespoon tamari or soy sauce

Cut off and discard the bottom 2-inch stem end of the bok choy. Separate the stems and rinse thoroughly under cool water. Drain on a kitchen towel. Cut the stems and the leaves on the diagonal into 1½-inch pieces. Spray a large skillet with nonstick cooking spray. Add the peanut oil. Tilt the skillet to coat with the oil and heat over medium heat. Add the garlic, almonds, ginger, and crushed red pepper. Cook for 3 minutes, stirring frequently, until the garlic is golden brown. Do not burn the garlic. Add the bok choy. Sprinkle lightly with salt and pepper. Cover and cook for about 20 minutes, stirring occasionally, until the stalks are tender to your preference. If the bok choy begins to stick, lower the heat to low-medium. When tender, stir in the tamari. Taste for seasonings.

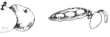

Broccoli with Garlic Chips

SERVES 6

My mom has turned us all into big fans of broccoli. She served this vitamin-packed vegetable in some delicious way just about every day while we were growing up. Broccoli and garlic, a traditional Italian combination, were just made for each other. The garlic chips take on a sharp, addictive flavor when you brown them in good olive oil. The chips are so tasty that sometimes they don't make it to the broccoli. I usually brown twice as much garlic as I really plan on adding to the broccoli—it's that delicious.

3 large stems of broccoli, with florets attached
3 tablespoons extra-virgin olive oil
8 large cloves garlic, thinly sliced lengthwise
　　Salt and pepper

Cut off and discard the bottom 1 inch of the broccoli stems. Peel the tough skin from the stems with a potato peeler. Cut each stem into thirds, keeping the florets intact. Bring a medium pot of lightly salted water to a boil. Cook the broccoli in the boiling water for 4 to 5 minutes until crisp-tender. Drain well. Rinse under cold water. Drain again. Arrange the broccoli on a serving platter. Set aside.

Heat the olive oil in a medium-size skillet over low-medium heat. Add the garlic slices and cook for about 5 minutes, stirring occasionally, until evenly browned. They should be a light to medium brown in color. Sprinkle with salt and pepper to taste. Pour the oil and garlic chips evenly over the broccoli. Taste for seasonings. Serve immediately or chilled.

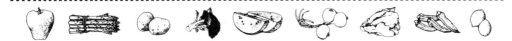

Brussels Sprouts in Lemon Vinaigrette

SERVES 6

I'm a big fan of brussels sprouts because of their crunch and their reputed health benefits. The touch of honey in this lemon vinaigrette makes these miniature members of the cabbage family even more enjoyable.

1 pound brussels sprouts
2 tablespoons walnut oil
1 large shallot, minced
1 tablespoon finely grated lemon zest
1 lemon, squeezed, about 2 tablespoons juice
2 tablespoons honey
  Salt and pepper

Trim the bottoms of the brussels sprouts, then carve a shallow X into the bottom of each with the tip of a small sharp knife. This will help them to cook evenly. Cook the brussels sprouts in lightly salted boiling water for about 10 minutes or until tender. Drain. In a skillet large enough to hold all the brussels sprouts, heat the oil over low-medium heat. Add the shallot and the lemon zest. Cook for 5 minutes, stirring occasionally, until the shallot is softened. Stir in the lemon juice, honey, and salt and pepper to taste. Add the drained brussels sprouts. Stir to coat. Cook for 2 minutes, stirring occasionally, until the sauce is heated through.

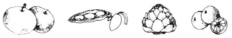

Sweet and Sour Red Cabbage

SERVES 8

This tangy, eastern European–style stew of red cabbage is the perfect accompaniment to veggie burgers. Add a tossed salad, or perhaps Natasha's Russian Salad from Minsk (page 56) and you will have a light dinner with the breezy feel of a picnic that you can enjoy any time of the year.

    3 tablespoons olive oil
    2 tablespoons soybean margarine (found in health food stores) or canola oil
    4 medium sweet onions, cut in half lengthwise, then crosswise into thick ribs
    1 large head red cabbage, cut into quarters, then cut into ½-inch slices
    1 28-ounce can Italian whole peeled tomatoes, with juice, crushed with your fingers
 1½ cups water
    ½ cup firmly packed brown sugar
    2 lemons, squeezed, about ⅓ cup juice
    ½ cup golden raisins
      Salt and pepper

Heat the oil and the margarine in a large pot over low-medium heat. Add the onions and the cabbage. Stir well to coat with oil. Cover and cook for 10 minutes, stirring occasionally, until the onions and cabbage are wilted. Add the tomatoes and water. Raise the heat to high. Stir well to combine. Cover and bring to a boil, stirring occasionally. When it reaches a boil, lower the heat to low-medium, and continue cooking at a low-medium boil for 1 hour, covered, stirring occasionally. Stir in the brown sugar, lemon juice, raisins, and salt and pepper to taste. Mix well to combine. Uncover, and continue cooking at a low-medium boil for 5 minutes, stirring occasionally. Taste for seasonings.

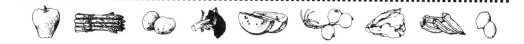

German-Style Red Cabbage and Apples

SERVES 6

My friend Lucy Bouck lives in a German neighborhood of St. Louis, Missouri. She has been a tremendous source of inspiration for me through our "food talks" and because of our mutual love for good food. She has shared many of her traditional German recipes with me, and this cabbage dish is a favorite.

- 3 tablespoons soybean margarine (found in health food stores) or canola oil
- 1 6-ounce package meatless bacon, cut into 1-inch pieces (found in supermarkets and health food stores)
- 1 large red (Bermuda) onion, cut in half, then thinly sliced
- 1 large head red cabbage, (about 3 pounds), quartered, then thinly sliced
- 1 medium Granny Smith apple, cored and cut into thin wedges
- 2 tablespoons firmly packed brown sugar
- 4 tablespoons apple cider vinegar
   Salt and pepper

Melt the margarine or heat the canola oil in a large pot over medium heat. Add the bacon, onion, cabbage, and apple. Mix well to coat, using tongs. Cover and cook for 20 minutes, stirring occasionally, until the cabbage is just tender. Stir in the brown sugar, vinegar, and salt and pepper to taste. Cover and continue cooking for 5 minutes, stirring occasionally. Taste for seasonings.

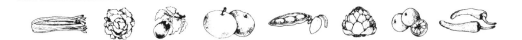

Savoy Cabbage Sautéed with Fresh Garlic

SERVES 6

My mother loves cabbage and cooks with it several times a week. Although she usually cooks delicious renditions of the many cabbage dishes her mother made while she was growing up, she occasionally experiments with the recipes she learned from Mrs. O'Keefe and Mrs. Funk, the Irish and Hungarian immigrant women she worked for when I was a young girl. This recipe combines the delicious flavors characteristic of Italian, Irish, and Hungarian cooking. I use savoy cabbage, a curly, pale green cabbage with a mild flavor. I serve this dish with Kasha with Sautéed Mushrooms and Onions (page 117) and Vegetable Burgers in an Orange-Mustard Sauce (page 181).

2 tablespoons soybean margarine (found in health food stores) or canola oil
1 tablespoon olive oil
2 cloves garlic, minced
1 medium red (Bermuda) onion, chopped
3 ounces Fakin' Bacon (found in health food stores) or other meatless bacon, chopped
1 medium savoy or green cabbage, cored and coarsely chopped
1 tablespoon caraway seeds
2 tablespoons paprika, preferably Hungarian
¼ cup water
   Salt and pepper

Heat the margarine and the olive oil in a large deep skillet or a large heavy pot over low heat. Add the garlic, onion, and meatless bacon. Cover and cook for 10 minutes, stirring occasionally. Add the cabbage. Sprinkle with the caraway seeds and the paprika. Add the water, and salt and pepper to taste. Raise the heat to medium. Cover and simmer for about 20 minutes, stirring occasionally, until the cabbage is tender. Taste for seasonings.

Orange-Maple Carrots

SERVES 6

You'll love the lively orange flavor in this recipe, and the maple syrup adds just the right amount of sweetness to this healthy, vitamin A-packed, fat-free side dish.

  8 medium carrots, peeled and cut on the diagonal in ½-inch slices
  1 cup orange juice (freshly squeezed if possible)
  ¼ cup pure maple syrup

Place all of the ingredients in a medium saucepan. Cover and bring to a boil over high heat, then lower the heat to medium. Cover and cook at a medium boil for about 10 minutes until the carrots are tender. Serve immediately or at room temperature.

Roasted Carrots with Dill

SERVES 6

The flavor combination of orange, dill, and sweet carrots is a knockout.

  6 large carrots, peeled and cut into 2-inch chunks
  ¼ cup orange juice (freshly squeezed if possible)
  2 tablespoons honey
  1½ teaspoons dried dillweed
      Salt and pepper

Preheat the oven to 375 degrees. Place the carrots, orange juice, honey, and dillweed in a bowl, and salt and pepper to taste. Toss well to mix. Spray a small baking dish with nonstick cooking spray. Turn the carrot mixture into the prepared baking dish. Cover tightly with foil. Bake for 35 minutes, until the carrots are tender when tested with a fork. Taste for seasonings.

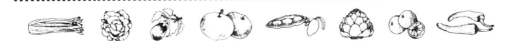

Sweet Cinnamon Carrots

SERVES 6

They look beautiful, smell wonderful, and taste delicious. They are rich in beta-carotene and are prepared without any fat. Maybe I should have named this luscious side dish Super Carrots!

  8 medium carrots, peeled and cut on the diagonal ¼-inch thick
  2 bay leaves
 ¼ cup firmly packed dark brown sugar
 ½ teaspoon cinnamon
  1 teaspoon pure vanilla extract
     Salt and pepper

Place the carrots in a small pot. Cover with cold water, then add an extra ½ inch of water. Add the bay leaves, brown sugar, cinnamon, and vanilla. Sprinkle lightly with salt and pepper and cover. Bring to a boil over high heat. Lower the heat to medium, remove the cover, and cook, uncovered, for about 5 minutes, stirring occasionally, until the carrots are fork-tender. Transfer the carrots from the cooking liquid to a serving bowl using a slotted spoon. Raise the heat under the cooking liquid to high and bring it to a boil. Lower the heat to low-medium and cook, uncovered, at a medium boil for about 30 minutes, stirring occasionally, until it reduces to a molasses-like consistency. Remove the bay leaves. Carefully taste for seasonings. Pour over the carrots. Serve immediately.

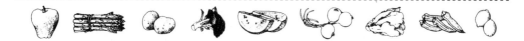

Italian-Style Sautéed Cauliflower

SERVES 6

One day at the supermarket, I came across the most beautiful head of pale orange cauliflower. Orange cauliflower (sometimes called pumpkin head cauliflower) has 6 times the amount of beta-carotene of regular white cauliflower! If you have an opportunity to buy one of these slightly sweet beauties for this recipe, please do.

- 3 tablespoons extra-virgin olive oil
- 3 large cloves garlic, minced
- 1 large head cauliflower, cored, stalks and florets coarsely chopped
- ¼ cup finely chopped fresh Italian flat-leaf parsley
- 5 basil leaves, coarsely chopped
  Salt and pepper
- 2 tablespoons water
- ¼ cup plain dry bread crumbs

Heat the olive oil in a large deep skillet over low-medium heat. Add the garlic, cauliflower, parsley, basil, and salt and pepper to taste. Cover and cook for about 35 minutes, stirring occasionally, until the cauliflower is just tender. Add the water and the bread crumbs. Stir to coat the cauliflower. Raise the heat to medium. Cover and continue cooking for 5 minutes, stirring occasionally. Taste for seasonings.

Parsleyed Cauliflower

SERVES 6

During that brief period when we thought potatoes were to blame for our weight-gain woes, I stopped eating them. My mother indulged me by making parsleyed cauliflower instead. Even though I'm back to eating potatoes (almost daily!), I still enjoy this delicious and oh so healthy side dish. Leftovers make a great addition to a frittata.

- 1 large head of cauliflower, green leaves discarded
- 3 tablespoons extra-virgin olive oil
- ¼ cup chopped fresh Italian flat-leaf parsley
  Salt and pepper

Cook the cauliflower in a covered pot of lightly salted boiling water for 15 to 20 minutes until it is fork-tender. Drain the cauliflower well. Set the cauliflower in a serving bowl. Drizzle the olive oil evenly over the cauliflower and scatter the chopped parsley on top. Sprinkle lightly with salt and pepper. Serve immediately.

Escarole Sautéed in Olive Oil with Garlic and Torn Bread

SERVES 6

My grandmother used to sauté her leftover escarole with lots of garlic and torn pieces of Italian bread. I like the combination so much that now I never wait for leftover escarole.

4 tablespoons extra-virgin olive oil
6 large cloves garlic, coarsely chopped
2 medium onions, cut in half, then into thin slices
1 teaspoon crushed red pepper
2 large heads escarole, coarsely chopped (about 2½ pounds)
  Salt and pepper
6 1-inch slices of Italian or French bread, torn into bite-size pieces

Heat the olive oil in a large, deep skillet over medium heat. Add the garlic, onions, and crushed red pepper. Cook for 5 minutes, stirring occasionally, until the onions have softened. Add the escarole. Sprinkle with salt and pepper to taste. Cover and cook for 15 minutes, stirring occasionally, until the escarole is tender. Add the bread. Stir to coat the bread. Cover and continue cooking for 5 to 7 minutes until the bread and escarole are soft. Taste for seasonings.

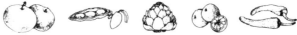

Corn with Lemon, Orange, and Thyme

SERVES 6

This is such a wonderful combination of flavors—sweet, herbal, citrusy, salty—that I could eat it every night.

2 tablespoons peanut oil
1 small sweet onion, finely chopped
1 tablespoon finely grated lemon zest
1 tablespoon finely grated orange zest
1 teaspoon dried thyme
  Salt and pepper
  Fresh corn kernels cut from 5 large ears of corn (about 5 cups)

In a large skillet, heat the peanut oil. Add the onion, lemon and orange zest, thyme, and salt and pepper to taste. Cover and cook for 2 minutes, stirring occasionally. Stir in the corn. Cover and cook for 6 minutes, stirring occasionally, until the corn is tender. Taste for seasonings.

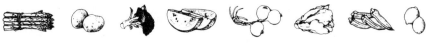

Stir-Fried Asian Vegetables

SERVES 6

Now that a wide variety of Asian vegetables is readily available in most super-markets, you can easily combine two or three vegetables for a delicious and healthy side dish.

 3 tablespoons peanut oil
 4 large cloves garlic, thinly sliced
 1 large head napa cabbage, coarsely chopped (about 2 pounds)
 ¼ pound shiitake mushrooms, stems removed and discarded, caps thinly sliced
 1 inch piece fresh gingerroot, peeled and finely minced
   Salt and white pepper
 ¼ pound snow peas, trimmed
 2 scallions, white part and 4 inches of green, cut into ½-inch slices
 2 tablespoons rice vinegar

Heat the peanut oil in a large deep skillet over medium heat. Add the garlic. Cook for 5 minutes, stirring frequently, until golden brown. Add the cabbage, mushrooms, gingerroot, and salt and pepper to taste. Cover and cook for 10 minutes, stirring occasionally, until the vegetables are crisp-tender. Stir in the snow peas, scallions, and the rice vinegar. Cook for 5 minutes, stirring occasionally. Taste for seasonings.

Maple-Glazed, Apple-Stuffed Acorn Squash

SERVES 4

We look forward to this delicious and abundantly healthy traditional New England side dish every fall and winter—it's even fat-free!

2 medium acorn squash, cut in half and seeded
2 large baking apples (Rome or Macintosh), cored and coarsely chopped
½ cup apple cider
4 tablespoons pure maple syrup
2 teaspoons cinnamon

Preheat oven to 450 degrees. Arrange the acorn squash, cut-side up, in a 9-inch glass baking dish. Spoon about one fourth of the apples into each cavity. Pour 2 tablespoons of the cider over each apple mound. Drizzle 1 tablespoon of the maple syrup over the apples and the cut side of each acorn squash. Sprinkle evenly with cinnamon. Pour 2 cups of water into the baking dish, around, not on the squash. Cover the dish tightly with foil, tenting as necessary. Bake for about 1 hour until the squash is tender when pierced with a fork.

Kale with Golden Raisins and Toasted Walnuts

SERVES 6

The addition of golden raisins and toasted walnuts along with a little balsamic vinegar give this vitamin- and calcium-packed side dish a lovely sweet taste.

    3 tablespoons olive oil
    3 large cloves garlic, minced
   ¼ cup chopped walnuts
    1 large bunch green kale, well washed and cut into 1-inch pieces
    3 tablespoons water
       Salt and pepper
   ½ cup golden raisins
    2 tablespoons sherry wine vinegar

Heat the olive oil in a large pot over medium heat. Add the garlic and walnuts. Cook for 5 minutes, stirring occasionally, until the garlic is golden brown. Add the kale, water, and salt and pepper to taste. Cover and cook for 20 minutes, stirring occasionally, until the kale is crisp-tender. Stir in the raisins, and the sherry vinegar. Continue cooking, uncovered, for 5 minutes. Taste for seasonings.

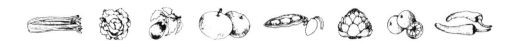

Portobello Mushrooms Sautéed with Olive Oil and Vermouth

SERVES 6

Big, brown portobello mushrooms have become a dinnertime favorite in both my restaurant and my home. I love their rich, meaty flavor and chewy texture and use them frequently in sauces, salads, and this luscious Italian side dish.

3 tablespoons extra-virgin olive oil
4 large cloves garlic, minced
1 large shallot, minced
8 ounces portobello mushroom caps, cut into ¼-inch slices
1 medium ripe tomato, diced
   Salt and pepper
3 tablespoons sweet vermouth

Heat the olive oil in a large skillet over medium heat. Add the garlic, shallot, mushrooms, and tomato. Sprinkle with salt and pepper to taste. Cover and cook for 7 to 10 minutes, stirring occasionally, until the mushrooms are just tender. Stir in the vermouth. Cook, uncovered, for 5 minutes, stirring occasionally. Taste for seasonings.

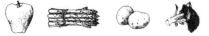

Onions Roasted with Herbs

SERVES 6

Roasted onions are wonderful with just about any entree, but I am partial to roasted onions served with Garlic Mashed Potatoes (page 105), gravy, and veggie burgers, plus Sautéed Spinach with Golden Raisins and Toasted Pine Nuts (page 109) and corn on the cob, for a family-style summer supper. Feel free to mix dried and fresh herbs or use all dried; this is one dish that always turns out wonderfully.

6 medium onions, cut in half lengthwise, then crosswise into thick ribs
2 tablespoons extra-virgin olive oil
1 teaspoon dried rosemary or 2 tablespoons fresh
½ teaspoon dried oregano or 2 teaspoons fresh
½ teaspoon dried basil or 2 teaspoons chopped fresh
½ teaspoon dried thyme or 2 teaspoons fresh
Salt and pepper

Preheat oven to 400 degrees. Place the onions in a large bowl. Drizzle the olive oil evenly over the onions. Toss to coat the onions, using two spoons. Sprinkle with rosemary, oregano, basil, thyme, and salt and pepper to taste over the onions. Toss thoroughly to coat evenly. Spray a 3-quart baking dish with nonstick cooking spray. Turn the onions into the prepared dish, using a rubber spatula to scrape the bowl. Cover the baking dish tightly with foil. Bake for 40 minutes, stirring once after 25 minutes, until the onions are tender.

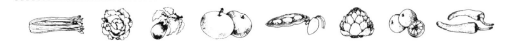

Gorgonzola-Stuffed Roasted Onions

SERVES 6

Jan Norris, the talented food editor of the Palm Beach Post, *told me about the stuffed whole onions that she wraps in foil and roasts over a campfire. Here is my indoor oven version.*

6 medium onions
4 ounces crumbled Gorgonzola cheese
1 tablespoon extra-virgin olive oil
1 teaspoon dried rosemary
1 teaspoon dried thyme
   Salt and pepper
1 cup water

Preheat the oven to 400 degrees. Peel the skin from the onions. Scoop out a hole about the width of a marble and 1 inch deep in the top of each onion, with a pointed teaspoon. Spray a baking dish with nonstick cooking spray. Arrange the onions with the holes facing up in the baking dish. Divide the Gorgonzola cheese among each onion, packing the cheese into the hole. Drizzle the olive oil evenly over the onions. Scatter the rosemary and thyme evenly over the onions. Sprinkle with salt and pepper to taste. Pour the water around, not over, the onions. Cover tightly with foil. Bake for 50 to 60 minutes, until the onions are fork-tender. Serve immediately.

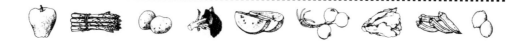

Mashed Parsnips, Sweet and White Potatoes

SERVES 6

My mother is truly the queen of vegetables. She steams and sautés, poaches and braises, roasts, fries, and mashes every vegetable that I know of. She was determined to get us to eat enough vegetables while growing up. Luckily, her great love of vegetables was passed on to me. With the wonderful combinations available to us year-round, it's no wonder that I don't have room on my plate for meat. Use any leftovers for Corn-Crusted Parsnip, Sweet and White Potato Cakes (page 252).

- 1 large parsnip, peeled and cut into 1-inch pieces
- 2 large sweet potatoes, peeled and cut into 2-inch pieces
- 6 large white potatoes, peeled and cut into 2-inch pieces
- ¼ cup reserved cooking liquid from the vegetables
- 2 tablespoons extra-virgin olive oil
- ¼ cup snipped fresh chives
    Salt and pepper

Cook the parsnip, sweet potatoes, and white potatoes in lightly salted boiling water for 12 to 15 minutes until soft-tender. Reserve ¼ cup cooking liquid. Drain well. Return the vegetables to the pot. Add the reserved cooking liquid. Mash together with a potato masher, until the mixture is still slightly lumpy. Add the olive oil, chives, and salt and pepper. Stir to mix. Taste for seasonings.

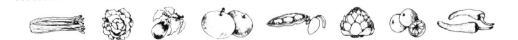

Garlic Mashed Potatoes

SERVES 6 OR 4 WITH LEFTOVERS FOR SHEPHERD'S PIE (PAGE 244)

We already know that when it comes to comfort food, just the sight of a bowl of beautiful, steaming mashed potatoes makes you feel happy. And the addition of aromatic slices of garlic, lightly fried in a fruity olive oil, is enough to send your tastebuds to heaven.

10 medium potatoes, peeled and quartered
   Salt
½ cup cooking liquid from the potatoes
 6 tablespoons soybean margarine or canola oil (found in health food stores)
½ cup soy milk
 2 tablespoons olive oil
 4 cloves garlic, sliced
   Freshly ground pepper

Place the potatoes in an 8-quart pot. Add cold water to cover potatoes, plus 3 inches. Sprinkle lightly with salt. Cover and bring to a boil over a high heat. Lower the heat to medium-high, and cook at a medium boil for about 12 minutes, until the potatoes are tender when pierced with a fork. Reserve ½ cup of the cooking liquid.

Drain the potatoes, then return them to the pot. Add the reserved cooking liquid and mash until smooth, using a potato masher. Stir in the soybean margarine, or canola oil, beating to combine. Add the soy milk. Beat well to combine. Set aside. Heat the olive oil in a small skillet over a medium heat. Add the garlic. Cook each side for about 1 to 2 minutes until golden brown. Add the browned garlic to the mashed potatoes. Stir to mix. Taste for seasonings.

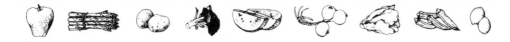

Scalloped Potatoes

SERVES 6

Rich, creamy, and scrumptious is how you will describe these luscious potatoes. But here are some other words for them: non-dairy, vegan, soy-enriched, and cholesterol-free.

7 medium potatoes
2 tablespoons extra-virgin olive oil
2 medium onions, cut in half lengthwise, then sliced thin
1 large shallot, minced
⅓ cup plus ¼ cup plain dry bread crumbs
2 cups soy milk
Salt and pepper

Peel the potatoes and slice them ¼-inch thick. As you slice the potatoes, place them in a bowl of lightly salted cool water. Preheat the oven to 400 degrees. Heat the olive oil in a skillet over medium heat. Add the onions and shallot. Cover and cook for about 25 minutes, stirring occasionally, until browned and caramelized. Add ⅓ cup of the bread crumbs and stir well to mix. Cook for 1 minute, stirring frequently. Gradually pour in the soy milk, stirring continuously as you pour. Cook for 10 minutes, stirring frequently. Stir in salt and pepper to taste.

Spray a 3-quart glass casserole dish with nonstick cooking spray. Ladle about ¼ cup of the onion mixture into the prepared dish. Drain the potatoes in a colander, then turn them into a bowl. Arrange about one third of the potatoes over the sauce in the dish. Ladle ¼ cup of sauce over the potatoes. Arrange the remaining potatoes over the sauce. Ladle the remaining sauce over the potatoes. Cover tightly with foil. Bake for about 1½ hours, or until the potatoes are tender when tested with a fork. When the potatoes are tender, sprinkle the remaining ¼ cup bread crumbs evenly over the potatoes. Continue baking, uncovered, for 10 minutes, until the potatoes are golden brown.

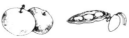

Mashed Sweet Potatoes

SERVES 4

Sweet potatoes are not just for the fall and winter months anymore. We always knew that they're delicious, and now we also know that they are powerhouses of beta-carotene. The brown sugar and pure maple syrup in this recipe add to the natural sweetness of the sweet potatoes for a real treat.

3 large sweet potatoes, peeled and quartered, then each quarter cut into
   4 pieces.
¼ stick (2 tablespoons) soybean margarine (found in health food stores) or
   canola oil
2 tablespoons firmly packed dark brown sugar
1 tablespoon pure maple syrup
   Salt and pepper

Cook the potatoes in lightly salted boiling water for about 15 minutes, until tender-soft. Drain. Return the potatoes to the cooking pot. Mash with a potato masher. Add the soy margarine. Continue mashing until the potatoes are as smooth as you like. Add the brown sugar and maple syrup. Sprinkle with salt and pepper to taste. Stir with the masher until the ingredients are mixed together. Taste for seasonings.

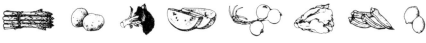

Candied Sweet Potatoes

SERVES 6

Sweet potatoes have always rated high with my family, right up there with healthy favorites like spinach and white potatoes. Although I can't think of any sweet potato dish that I don't care for, this remains my favorite recipe.

3 tablespoons soybean margarine (found in health food stores) or butter
3 large sweet potatoes, peeled and cut into 1-inch rounds
1 cup water
½ cup firmly packed dark brown sugar
1 tablespoon ground cinnamon
1 tablespoon pure vanilla extract
  Salt

Melt the margarine in a medium skillet (with 2- to 3-inch-high sides) over low-medium heat. Add the sweet potatoes, fitting as many as you can in a single layer. Then arrange another layer over the first layer. Pour the water evenly over the potatoes. Sprinkle the brown sugar and cinnamon evenly over the potatoes. Drizzle the vanilla evenly over the potatoes. Sprinkle lightly with salt. Cover the skillet and cook over low-medium heat at a low-medium boil for 25 minutes without stirring. Turn the potatoes over, rotating the top layer to the bottom, turning those potatoes over as well to cook the other side. Keep in mind while turning that both sides of each slice need a turn on the bottom in the center of the skillet, to caramelize properly. Cover and continue to cook for about 15 minutes, turning the potatoes over to coat with the syrupy cooking liquid until the potatoes are tender when tested with a fork.

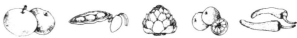

Sautéed Spinach with Golden Raisins and Toasted Pine Nuts

SERVES 4

My grandmother often added raisins and pine nuts (pignoli) to her meatballs, stuffing, and this delicious sautéed spinach recipe. This traditional Sicilian side dish makes a great pasta dish, too—simply add cooked linguine (or any pasta) to the skillet of sautéed spinach and toss together.

3 tablespoons extra-virgin olive oil
5 large cloves garlic, coarsely chopped
1 teaspoon crushed red pepper
1 10-ounce bag spinach, thoroughly rinsed and well drained
2 tablespoons golden raisins
3 tablespoons toasted pine nuts (see Note)
  Salt and pepper

Heat oil in a large skillet over low-medium heat. Add the garlic and crushed red pepper. Cook for 2 to 3 minutes, stirring frequently, until the garlic is just golden brown. Add the spinach (don't worry if it's a big mound, it will shrink down). Cover the skillet, or rest the cover on the mound of spinach.

After 3 to 4 minutes, when the spinach shrinks down, stir to mix. I find it helpful to use tongs to turn the spinach. Add the raisins and pine nuts. Sprinkle with salt and pepper to taste. Stir to mix. Cook, uncovered, for 3 to 4 minutes, stirring occasionally until the spinach is cooked to your liking. Taste for seasonings.

NOTE: To toast the pine nuts, preheat your oven to 400 degrees. Spread the pine nuts in a pie dish. Bake for about 5 minutes or until golden brown. You'll want a taste, but be careful to wait a minute—the nuts don't look it, but they are very hot.

Spinach and Leeks in Pernod

SERVES 4

Pernod is a licorice-flavored liqueur and a little bit of it works wonderfully with spinach.

    3 tablespoons olive oil
    1 large leek, white part and 8 inches of green, coarsely chopped
    1 10-ounce bag spinach, well washed and coarsely chopped
    1 large tomato, diced
      Salt and pepper
    ¼ cup Pernod

Heat the oil in a medium pot over medium heat. Add the leek, spinach, and tomato. Sprinkle with salt and pepper to taste. Cover and cook for about 12 minutes, stirring occasionally, until the leeks are crisp-tender. Stir in the Pernod. Cook, uncovered, for 5 minutes, stirring occasionally. Taste for seasonings.

Roasted Fennel and Tomatoes

SERVES 8

My mom roasted fennel along with tomatoes, onions, and sausages for a one-dish dinner entree. In this side dish, the lemon juice adds a nice zip to a delicious combination.

    1 large head fennel, cut in half lengthwise, then crosswise into 1-inch ribs
    3 large ripe tomatoes, cut into 1-inch wedges
    1 medium onion, cut in half lengthwise, then crosswise into ½-inch ribs
    2 tablespoons extra-virgin olive oil
    1 lemon, squeezed about 3 tablespoons juice
      Salt and pepper

Preheat oven to 350 degrees. Place the fennel, tomatoes, and onion in a bowl. Add the olive oil and lemon juice. Toss well to coat. Add salt and pepper to taste. Spray a baking pan with nonstick cooking spray. Turn the fennel mixture into the prepared pan. Bake for 1 hour, stirring once to mix, until the fennel is tender-crisp.

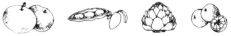

Herbed Barley with Almonds

SERVES 6

I love plain barley with a little butter on top as a side dish, sometimes in place of rice. It's a delicious change and also a good source of fiber. Here's a more flavorful, fragrant dish that's great with many vegetable entrees.

- 1 pound barley
- 3 tablespoons soybean margarine (found in health food stores), cut into thin slices, or canola oil
- 1 large shallot, minced
- ¼ cup slivered almonds
- 8 to 10 large fresh basil leaves
  Salt and pepper

Bring 4 quarts of lightly salted water to a boil in a large covered pot over high heat. Stir in the barley. Lower the heat to medium. Cook for about 1 hour, stirring occasionally, until tender. Drain. Return the barley to the pot. Add the margarine, shallot, almonds, basil leaves, and salt and pepper to taste. Stir well to mix and to melt the margarine, if using. Taste for seasonings.

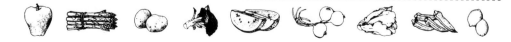

Sautéed Zucchini Spears

SERVES 8

You can enjoy this traditional Italian side dish with almost any dinner, or eat them as a snack, as part of an antipasto platter, or as a sandwich filling with just a squeeze of lemon juice on top. They make the perfect accompaniment to a glass of wine before your evening meal.

4 medium zucchini
Salt
3 tablespoons extra virgin olive oil
4 large cloves garlic, sliced lengthwise
2 large shallots, coarsely chopped
Pepper

Cut each zucchini in half lengthwise, then in half crosswise, then cut each quarter into 4 spears. Place the zucchini spears in a large colander. Sprinkle liberally with salt. Toss well to coat. Set aside for 10 minutes, tossing occasionally. Spray a large skillet with nonstick cooking spray. Heat the skillet over a medium-high heat. Spread 1 tablespoon of olive oil evenly over the bottom of the skillet, using a pastry brush. Arrange as many zucchini spears as you can fit, cut-side down, in a single layer in the skillet. Cook each side for about 5 minutes, until lightly browned, using tongs to turn the spears. Transfer the browned spears to a serving platter. Repeat the process until all of the zucchini spears are browned. Spray the skillet again. Scatter the garlic and the shallots in the skillet. Sprinkle with salt and pepper to taste. Cook for about 3 minutes, stirring occasionally, until golden brown. Scatter the browned garlic and shallots evenly over the sautéed zucchini spears. Serve immediately or slightly chilled.

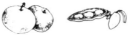

Refried Black Beans

SERVES 8

All of the flavor of Mexican refried beans, yet none of the cholesterol! This is my kind of dish. The rich smoky flavor in this recipe comes from meatless bacon. I use Fakin' Bacon, made by LightLife Foods, found in most health food stores. Some supermarkets sell other brands of meatless bacon, so do try different brands and use your favorite. Serve with Corn-Crusted Parsnip, Sweet and White Potato Cakes (page 252) and Avocado, Tomato, and Onion Salad (page 33).

12 ounces black turtle beans, picked over for stones
 3 tablespoons olive oil
 3 ounces meatless bacon, chopped
 1 medium yellow onion, finely chopped
 1 large clove garlic, minced
 1 teaspoon ground cumin
   Salt and pepper
¾ cup reserved cooking liquid from the beans

Place the beans in a large pot. Add 3 quarts of water. Cover. Bring to a boil over high heat. Lower the heat to medium. Cover and cook at a medium boil for about 1½ hours, stirring occasionally, until the beans are soft. Reserve ¾ cup of cooking liquid. Drain the beans. Set aside. Heat the oil in a large skillet over medium heat. Add the meatless bacon, onion, and garlic. Cover and cook for 10 minutes, stirring occasionally, until the onions are softened and have released their juices. Add the drained beans. Sprinkle with the cumin, and salt and pepper to taste. Add the reserved cooking liquid. Mash the beans with a potato masher until they are creamy and somewhat smooth. Taste for seasonings.

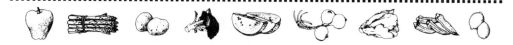

White Beans Stewed with Tomatoes and Sage

SERVES 8

This flavorful combination is delicious and rich in fiber and protein and it has tremendous versatility. You can serve it as a side dish with any Italian meal, it makes a fine topping for Fresh Corn Polenta with Tomatoes and Basil Ricotta (page 115), or you can toss it over your favorite pasta for an easy and healthy dinner. This fragrant stew is also a wonderful topping for pizza.

  1 pound dried cannellini beans (white kidney beans) or great northern
    beans, picked over for stones
  3 tablespoons extra-virgin olive oil
  2 large cloves garlic, minced
  4 medium tomatoes, chopped, juices included
 12 fresh sage leaves, chopped
  1 teaspoon dried sage
    Salt and pepper

Place beans in a large heavy pot. Add 2 quarts of water. Cover and bring to a boil over high heat. Lower the heat to low-medium. Cook, covered, at a low-medium boil for 1 hour, stirring occasionally. Continue cooking, uncovered, for 45 minutes, stirring occasionally, until the beans are soft. Lower the heat if the beans begin to stick. Meanwhile, heat the olive oil in a large skillet over low-medium heat. Add the garlic and tomatoes with their juices. Cook, uncovered, for 5 minutes, stirring occasionally. Stir in the sage leaves and dried sage. Sprinkle with salt and pepper to taste. Continue cooking for 20 minutes, stirring occasionally, until the tomatoes are soft. Set aside. When the beans are soft, add the sautéed tomato mixture. Stir well to combine. Adjust seasonings, adding more salt if necessary. Cook for 2 minutes, stirring occasionally. Taste for seasonings.

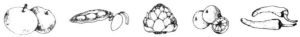

Fresh Corn Polenta with Tomatoes and Basil Ricotta

SERVES 6

My grandmother always made large quantities of polenta, a traditional Italian favorite, so that she could have enough for the next day's breakfast. She cut the leftover polenta into squares, then fried the squares in a little butter and sprinkled the polenta with grated Parmesan cheese. Now that's a wonderful way to start a day! This polenta is perfectly delicious with or without the basil ricotta.

9 cups water
  Fresh corn kernels cut from 1 to 2 large ears of corn (about 1½ cups)
1 medium tomato, finely chopped, including juices
3 cups cornmeal
  Salt and pepper
1 cup ricotta cheese
¼ cup finely chopped fresh basil leaves

Bring the water to a boil in a large covered pot. Stir in the corn kernels and the tomato. Cook, uncovered, at a rapid boil for 2 minutes, stirring occasionally. Put on oven mitts to protect your hands from burning while you proceed with the recipe. Whisking continuously, gradually pour the cornmeal into the boiling liquid in a steady stream. Be careful of the bubbling mixture. Sprinkle with salt and pepper to taste. Lower the heat to medium. Continue cooking at a medium-high boil for 5 minutes, whisking frequently. Remove from heat, taste for seasonings.

Spoon the ricotta into a serving bowl. Add the basil. Stir together to mix. Pour the polenta onto a large serving platter. Top each serving of polenta with a spoonful of the basil-ricotta mixture.

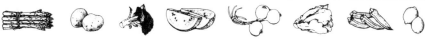

Fresh Corn-Cilantro Cornbread

SERVES 6 TO 8

I can't think of anything better to serve with Mexican-inspired foods than this delicious, soy-enriched cornbread. Candied Sweet Potatoes (page 108) with this cornbread and a salad make a great picnic.

- 2 eggs or equivalent egg substitute
- 1 cup soy milk
- 2 tablespoons unsweetened applesauce
- 2 tablespoons peanut oil
- 1 cup unbleached white flour
- 3 tablespoons firmly packed dark brown sugar
- 1½ cups cornmeal
- 1 teaspoon baking powder
- 1 cup fresh corn kernels, cut from 2 ears, *or* 1 cup frozen corn
- 2 tablespoons chopped cilantro

Preheat oven to 425 degrees. Place the eggs in a mixing bowl. Whisk together for 10 seconds or until blended. Add the remaining ingredients. Whisk together for about 15 seconds until combined. Spray a 10-inch glass pie pan with cooking spray. Pour the batter into the prepared pan, using a rubber spatula to scrape the bowl and then to smooth the top of the batter evenly. Bake on the center rack of the oven for about 25 minutes, until a cake tester comes out clean when inserted into the center. Cut into wedges and serve warm, either plain or with soybean margarine.

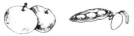

Kasha with Sautéed Mushrooms and Onions

SERVES 8

Kasha, a longtime Russian staple made from buckwheat kernels, is readily available in supermarkets. It has a terrific, nutty flavor and a lot of fiber, too. Try serving this hearty kasha any time you would ordinarily serve rice or potatoes. I prefer to use shiitake or button mushrooms and Vidalia onions in this recipe.

- 2 tablespoons soybean margarine (found in health food stores) or canola oil
- 1 tablespoon extra-virgin olive oil
- 1 large sweet onion, finely chopped
- 1 pound mushrooms, cut in ¼-inch slices
- 5 cups water
- 2 cups kasha
- Salt and pepper

Melt the margarine or heat the oil in a medium pot over low-medium heat. Add the olive oil. Heat for 1 minute. Add the onion and mushrooms. Cover and cook for 10 minutes, stirring occasionally. Add the water. Raise heat to high. When the water comes to a boil, lower heat to low-medium. Add the kasha, and salt and pepper to taste. Stir well to mix. Cover and cook at a low-medium boil for about 25 minutes, stirring occasionally, until the kasha is tender. Taste for seasonings.

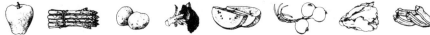

Matzo Brei

SERVES 6

Matzo is an unleavened bread traditionally eaten during the Jewish holiday of Passover, but it's available year-round. When Ed Portnoy gave me the recipe for his family's favorite matzo brei, he told me: "My grandmother from Austria made it, my mother made it, and now I make it." You can eat matzo brei for breakfast with salt and pepper or sugar and jam, or as a side dish with a dinner of Kasha with Cabbage and Portobello Mushrooms (page 257) and Sweet Cinnamon Carrots (page 93). Enjoy this recipe and pass it on to the next generation.

10 matzos (1 10-ounce box) found in the import or kosher section of most supermarkets
 3 cups hot tap water
10 eggs or equivalent egg substitute
½ cup plus 2 tablespoons soy milk or low-fat milk
    Salt and pepper
 1 tablespoon soybean margarine (found in health food stores) or canola oil

Break the matzos into bite-size pieces and place in a large bowl. Pour the hot water evenly over the matzos. Stir the matzos, pressing lightly with the back of a wooden spoon to allow them to absorb the hot water. Turn into a colander and drain, using a wooden spoon to gently press out the water. In a separate bowl, lightly beat the eggs with a whisk. Whisk in the soy milk, and salt and pepper to taste, and continue whisking until it is well blended. Pour this over the matzos and stir to mix. Melt the margarine in a large, nonstick skillet over medium heat. Pour in the matzo mixture, using a rubber spatula to scrape the bowl. Cover and cook for about 20 minutes, stirring occasionally, until the eggs are fully cooked. Taste for seasonings.

Basmati Rice with Green Peas and Pine Nuts

SERVES 8

Basmati rice, grown in the Himalayas for thousands of years, is one of many in-teresting varieties of rice available in our supermarkets today. It has a delicate, nutty flavor. I love to serve this rice with a curried dish, although it also adds a special flavor to bean soups. It is always a pleasant alternative to white or plain brown rice.

     2 tablespoons peanut oil
     ½ medium red (Bermuda) onion, finely chopped
     1 teaspoon curry powder
       Salt and pepper
    14 ounces basmati rice (about 2 cups)
     ¼ cup apple juice
    1¾ cups water
     1 cup frozen green peas, defrosted
     ¼ cup pine nuts

Heat the oil in a large skillet over medium-high heat. Add the onion. Sprinkle with curry powder, and salt and pepper to taste. Cook for 3 minutes, stirring oc-casionally. Add the rice, stirring to coat. Cook for 1 minute, stirring occasionally. Stir in the apple juice, mixing well to combine. Stir in the water. Cover and lower the heat to medium-low. Simmer, covered, for about 40 minutes until the rice is tender and the liquid is absorbed. Stir in the green peas and the pine nuts. Taste for seasonings.

Basmati Rice Pilaf

SERVES 6

My first experience with this tasty rice was in Indian restaurants—its fragrance is wonderful with curry dishes. Now I often serve this rice in place of plain brown or white rice, both at home and at Claire's.

2 tablespoons peanut oil
1 medium onion, finely chopped
1 medium carrot, peeled and finely diced
1 small zucchini, finely diced
¼ cup pine nuts
1 14-ounce box basmati rice, about 2 cups
5 cups water
  Salt and pepper

Heat the oil in a medium pot over medium heat. Add the onion, carrot, zucchini, and pine nuts. Cook for 5 minutes, uncovered, stirring occasionally, until the onions are softened. Stir in the rice. Add the water, and salt and pepper to taste. Stir well to mix. Cover. Raise the heat to high and bring to a boil. Lower the heat to low-medium. Cook, covered, at a low boil for 35 to 40 minutes until tender. Taste for seasonings.

Leban (Lebanese Yogurt)

MAKES ABOUT 16 CUPS

Once you see just how easy (and delicious) homemade yogurt is to make, you may never buy it again. You don't even need any special equipment—your finger is the best thermometer! This recipe produces the smoothest and creamiest yogurt I've ever had. It was bestowed on me by a Lebanese woman named Sadie Saba, who came over one day to share recipes while visiting her daughter Mary Lou. Sadie was thrilled to share her recipes with a "young woman of the newer generation" who was still interested in cooking. She soon learned that my life revolves around food! Serve it plain, topped with fresh fruit, or use as you would other yogurt.

  1 gallon whole milk
⅔ cup plain, whole milk yogurt

Heat the milk in a large, uncovered pot over medium heat, without stirring, until it begins to foam up. When the foam reaches about halfway to the top of the pan, remove from the heat. Pour the heated milk into a large bowl (a tempered glass or pottery bowl is best). Set the bowl on your counter to cool until you can insert your smallest finger into the center of the bowl of milk comfortably for 10 full seconds. Measure the yogurt into a separate bowl. Add 6 tablespoons of the heated milk to the bowl of yogurt. Stir well to mix. Pour the yogurt mixture into the large bowl of heated milk, using a rubber spatula to scrape the bowl clean. (This is the point when Sadie said a blessing over the bowl.)

Cover the bowl with a plate large enough to fit over the bowl without touching the yogurt. Cover the bowl with a clean dish towel, then a thick bath towel. Leave the wrapped bowl on the counter for 8 hours, without disturbing. After 8 hours, remove the towels but leave the plate on. Refrigerate for 8 hours. Remove from the refrigerator, remove about ¾ cup of the top layer and spoon this into a jar. Cover the jar and refrigerate for up to two weeks. This will be your yogurt "starter" for your next batch. You may now begin eating and enjoying your homemade yogurt.

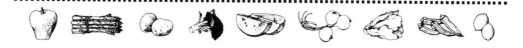

Tequila-Lime Sauce

MAKES ABOUT 1 CUP

The snappy flavor of tequila and fresh lime in this mayonnaise-based sauce is the perfect accompaniment to Corn-Crusted Parsnip, Sweet and White Potato Cakes (page 252). You can also enjoy this delicious, Mexican-inspired sauce as a dip for raw vegetables, and it's excellent on baked potatoes, too. Prepare a large batch and use it as a dressing for a pasta or potato salad.

¼ cup dairy-free mayonnaise (found in health food stores)
1 tablespoon finely grated lime zest
2 limes, squeezed, about 3 tablespoons juice
1 tablespoon chopped fresh Italian flat-leaf parsley
1 tablespoon chopped fresh cilantro
2 large cloves garlic, chopped
1 tablespoon tequila
2 tablespoons soy milk
  Salt and pepper

Place all of the ingredients in a blender. Cover. Pulse the mixture 5 to 6 times. Stop and scrape the sides down, using a rubber spatula. Cover and pulse another 4 to 5 times until the mixture is well blended. Taste for seasonings. Stir and serve. Can be refrigerated up to 3 days.

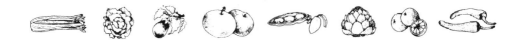

Portobello and Cremini Mushroom and Herb Gravy

MAKES ABOUT 2½ CUPS

The portobello mushrooms have a rich, meaty texture and the cremini mushrooms lend an earthy flavor to this lovely gravy. Is there any greater comfort than eating a bowl of steaming Garlic Mashed Potatoes (page 105) covered with gravy?

  2 tablespoons extra-virgin olive oil
  2 tablespoons soybean margarine (found in health food stores)
  1 small sweet onion, chopped
10 medium cremini mushrooms, sliced
  2 medium portobello mushrooms, trimmed and chopped
  1 teaspoon dried thyme
  1 teaspoon dried sage
    Salt and pepper
  3 cups water
  4 tablespoons cornstarch
  1 tablespoon Grand Marnier

Measure the oil and soybean margarine into a 12-inch skillet. Add the onion and cook over a low-medium heat for 4 minutes, stirring occasionally until the onions have softened. Add the mushrooms. Sprinkle with the thyme, sage, salt, and pepper. Cover and cook for 5 minutes, stirring frequently, until the mushrooms are barely tender. In a bowl, whisk together the water and cornstarch. Add this mixture to the mushrooms. Stir well to mix. Raise the heat to medium-high and bring the mixture to a boil, stirring frequently. Lower the heat to medium. Cook at a low-medium boil, uncovered, for 10 to 12 minutes, stirring frequently, until thickened. Stir in the Grand Marnier. Taste for seasonings.

Cranberry-Lime Sauce

MAKES ABOUT 2¼ CUPS

Cranberries are native to North America and they make a tangy sauce that is a perfect accompaniment to stuffed acorn squash. I also love this cranberry sauce alongside Garlic Mashed Potatoes (page 105) and Portobello and Cremini Mushroom and Herb Gravy (page 123), too. And cranberries are rich in vitamin C and fiber, so you can feel good about taking a second helping.

12 ounces fresh, whole cranberries
¾ cup sugar
½ cup orange juice (freshly squeezed if possible)
⅓ cup water
 1 teaspoon grated lime zest
 1 lime, squeezed, about 2 tablespoons juice

Place all ingredients in a 4-quart pot. Stir to mix. Cover and bring to a boil over a high heat. Lower heat to low-medium and cook at a low-medium boil for 10 minutes, stirring frequently. Turn into a bowl. Serve immediately or cool to room temperature. Can be refrigerated for up to one week.

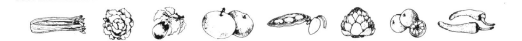

Sawmill Gravy

MAKES 2½ CUPS

I discovered sawmill gravy during a barbecue in San Antonio, Texas. The aroma was wonderful, but the gravy was off limits for my vegetarian diet. Luckily, the young woman sharing my table was a native Texan who told me just what went into the gravy. Within a couple of weeks, I was savoring my luscious vegetarian version back at home. Serve this gravy over Biscuits (page 126) and Chicken-Fried Vegetable Burgers (page 183).

- 3 tablespoons extra-virgin olive oil
- 6 ounces meatless sausage, crumbled (found in health food stores)
- 3 tablespoons flour
- 3 cups soy milk
  Salt and pepper

Heat the olive oil in a large skillet over medium heat. Add the sausage. Cook for about 5 minutes, stirring frequently, until browned. Sprinkle the flour evenly over the sausage. Stir well to coat evenly. Cook for about 3 minutes, stirring frequently with a wooden spoon, scraping the bottom of the pan as you stir. Gradually pour in the soy milk, stirring continuously as you pour. Continue stirring until the mixture is well blended. Stir in salt and pepper to taste. Lower the heat to medium-low, and cook at a simmer for about 30 minutes, stirring frequently, until the gravy has thickened. Taste for seasonings.

Biscuits

MAKES 12 BISCUITS

My husband loves the biscuits and gravy that all the restaurants seem to serve on our annual drive south. His chicken-based biscuits and gravy always smell so wonderful that I knew I needed to make a vegetarian version for myself. I adapted a recipe I got from a "born and raised" Texan I met in San Antonio, Texas. There's a lot to be said for necessity being the mother of invention. Enjoy!

- 2 cups flour
- 2 teaspoons baking powder
- ¼ teaspoon salt
- ¼ cup Spectrum spread (this is a nonhydrogenated vegetable shortening found in health food stores)
- ¾ cup soy milk

Preheat the oven to 425 degrees. Measure the flour, baking powder, and salt into a bowl, then sift it into another bowl. Add the Spectrum spread. Use two butter knives to cut the spread into the flour until it resembles coarse cornmeal. Gradually add the soy milk, stirring as you pour. Stir to mix into a sticky dough. Spray a cookie sheet with nonstick cooking spray. Drop the dough by heaping teaspoonfuls onto the prepared cookie sheet in rows. You should have room for 4 rows of 3 biscuits, about 1 inch apart from each other. Bake for about 15 minutes until golden brown and a cake tester comes out clean when inserted into the center of a biscuit.

4
Pastas and Sauces

- Linguine with Sautéed Zucchini Spears
- Angel Hair Pasta with Spinach, Tomatoes, Leeks, and Goat Cheese
- Farfalle with Garlic-Roasted Eggplant in Creamy Spinach Sauce
- Fettuccine with Sautéed Onions, Meatless Bacon, and Green Peas in Lemon Sauce
- Farfalle with Peppers, Artichoke Hearts, and Capers in White Wine Sauce
- Fettuccine in Vodka Sauce with Garden Vegetables and "Sausage"
- Linguine with Leeks, Red Onion, Carrots, Broccoli, and Asparagus
- Linguine with Artichoke Hearts, Tomatoes, and Leeks
- Farfalle with Tomatoes and Swiss Chard
- Orzo with Oven-Roasted Vegetables
- Noodles and Mushrooms in Creamy Sherry Sauce
- Pappardelle with Shiitake, Cremini, and Button Mushroom Sauce
- Pappardelle with Vegetable Cacciatore
- Penne with Roasted Potatoes, Onions, and Green Peas in Lemon-Wine Sauce
- Penne with San Marzano Tomatoes, Shiitake Mushrooms, Leeks, and Vermouth
- Penne with Tofu Sausage, Mushrooms, Black Olives, and Peperoncini in Marsala Wine Sauce
- Rigatoni with Tomatoes, Mushrooms, Pernod, and Goat Cheese
- Rigatoni with Green Beans and Tomatoes
- Pasta Puttanesca
- Rigatoni with "Sausages," Mushrooms, and Italian-Style Tofu
- Rigatoni with Mushrooms in a Creamy Whisky Sauce

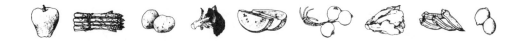

- Sesame Noodles
- Tortellini in Creamy Tomato Sauce with Artichoke Hearts
- Linguine with Extra-Virgin Olive Oil, Garlic, and Walnuts
- Ziti with Escarole, Potatoes, and Sun-Dried Tomatoes
- Ziti with Fava Beans and Dandelion Greens
- Broccoli Rabe Lasagna
- Pumpkin Squash Lasagna
- Hearty Bell Pepper-"Bacon" Sauce over Gnocchi
- Tortellini with Green Peas, Red Onion, and Meatless Bacon
- Spicy Fresh Tomato and "Cream"-Sauced Penne
- Meatless Bolognese Sauce for Rigatoni
- Marinara Sauce

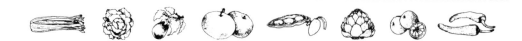

Linguine with Sautéed Zucchini Spears

SERVES 6

*My mother has always taken the city bus to work at **Claire's**. She doesn't drive, even though I've arranged for professional driving lessons for her. She claims that learning how to drive is "just too much." Well, I have another theory. I think my mother rides the city bus because it gives her the opportunity to pass recipes back and forth—that's where she got this one. I bet she's known how to drive all along!*

- ¼ cup extra-virgin olive oil
- 6 large cloves garlic, coarsely chopped
- 2 medium sweet onions, thinly sliced
- 4 medium zucchini (about 2 pounds), halved crosswise and then quartered lengthwise into spears
- 10 large basil leaves
  Salt and pepper
- 1 pound linguine
- 1 cup reserved cooking liquid from the linguine
  Freshly grated Parmesan cheese (optional)

Heat the olive oil in a large deep pot over medium heat. Add the garlic and the onions. Cook for 15 minutes, stirring occasionally, until the onions are golden brown. Add the zucchini and the basil leaves. Stir in salt and pepper to taste. Stir well to coat evenly. Cover and cook for 20 minutes, stirring occasionally until the zucchini are crisp-tender.

Meanwhile, cook the linguine according to package directions, reserving 1 cup of the cooking liquid just before draining. When the zucchini are crisp-tender, stir in the reserved cooking liquid from the pasta. Cover and continue cooking for about 5 minutes, or until the zucchini are just tender. Add the drained linguine. Toss well to coat the linguine evenly, using two spoons. Taste for seasonings. Turn into a serving bowl. Serve with freshly grated Parmesan cheese, if desired.

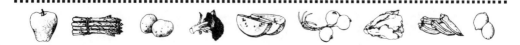

Angel Hair Pasta with Spinach, Tomatoes, Leeks, and Goat Cheese

SERVES 6 TO 8

When I first cooked this lovely sauce, my recipe did not include any goat cheese, and it was perfectly delicious. But when I stirred some goat cheese into the sauce just before serving (at my husband Frank's suggestion) the flavor was exquisite! The goat cheese adds a light creaminess and a rich, earthy flavor to the dish. We've made this sauce with many varieties (and degrees of firmness) of goat cheese and each brand has lent its own interesting flavor.

    3 tablespoons extra-virgin olive oil
    2 large shallots, finely chopped
    ½ small red (Bermuda) onion, finely chopped
    4 large cloves garlic, finely chopped
    1 large leek, white part and 2 inches of pale green, coarsely chopped
    5 large ripe tomatoes, chopped
    ¼ cup finely chopped fresh Italian flat-leaf parsley
    ¼ cup dry white wine
      Salt and pepper
    1 10-ounce bag spinach, well rinsed and drained, coarsely chopped
   10 to 12 fresh basil leaves
    4 ounces goat cheese, crumbled
    1 pound angel hair pasta (capellini)

Put the water on to boil for your pasta while you prepare the sauce. Spray a large deep skillet with nonstick cooking spray. Add the olive oil. Heat over medium heat. Add the shallots, red onion, garlic, and leek. Cook for 5 minutes, stirring occasionally, until the onion and leeks have softened and released some of their liquids. Add the tomatoes, parsley, and wine. Sprinkle with salt and pepper to taste. Stir well to mix. Cook for about 12 minutes, stirring occasionally, as the sauce cooks at a low-medium boil. Add the spinach and basil leaves. Continue cooking at a low-medium boil for another 10 minutes, stirring frequently, until the tomatoes are soft and the spinach is tender. Stir in the goat cheese, mixing well to combine. Continue cooking for 1 minute, stirring occasionally, until the cheese melts into the sauce. Taste for seasonings. Cover and remove from heat. Cook the pasta according to the package directions. Drain well. Return the pasta to the pot. Ladle two thirds of the sauce over the pasta. Toss well using two spoons to coat the pasta evenly. Add the remaining sauce and toss well. Turn into a warm serving bowl. Serve immediately.

Farfalle with Garlic-Roasted Eggplant in Creamy Spinach Sauce

SERVES 6 TO 8

Eggplant and spinach have been mainstay vegetables at home and at **Claire's** *for as long as I can remember, and when you combine the two, adding garlic and a light creamy sauce, the results are "awesome"—as my nephew Branden says.*

- 2 medium eggplants (do not peel), cut into 1-inch cubes
  Salt
- 6 large cloves garlic, finely chopped
- 4 tablespoons extra-virgin olive oil
- 2 tablespoons water
- 2 teaspoons dried oregano
- 1 10-ounce bag spinach, washed well and coarsely chopped
- ¼ cup coarsely chopped fresh Italian flat-leaf parsley
- ½ teaspoon crushed red pepper
  Pepper
- 2 cups soy milk (found in most supermarkets and in health food stores)
- 1 pound farfalle pasta (bow ties)

Preheat oven to 400 degrees. Place the cubed eggplant in a large bowl. Sprinkle generously with salt. Toss well to coat. Add half of the chopped garlic. Toss well. Add 2 tablespoons of the olive oil, and toss well to coat the cubes evenly. Sprinkle the water over the top and toss well to coat. Sprinkle the oregano over the top and toss well to coat. Spray a large roasting pan with nonstick cooking spray. Turn the eggplant into the prepared pan, spreading evenly. Cover tightly with foil. Bake on the bottom rack of the oven for 35 to 40 minutes, stirring once, until the eggplant is soft. After you stir the eggplant rotate the pan on the rack so that the eggplant will cook more evenly.

Meanwhile, heat the remaining 2 tablespoons of olive oil in a large pot over medium heat. Add the remaining garlic and cook for 3 minutes, stirring occasion-

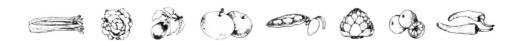

ally, until softened. Add the spinach, parsley, and crushed red pepper. Sprinkle lightly with salt and pepper. Cover and cook for 6 to 8 minutes, stirring frequently, until the spinach is tender. Stir in the soy milk, mixing well to combine. Cover and cook for 5 minutes, stirring occasionally.

Meanwhile, cook the pasta according to package directions and drain well. Remove the sauce from the heat and keep covered. When the eggplant is cooked, add the eggplant and the pan juices to the pot of spinach. Place the pot over medium heat, cover, and cook for 2 minutes, stirring occasionally. Add the cooked and drained farfalle pasta to the pot. Stir well to mix. Cover and cook for 3 minutes, stirring occasionally. Taste for seasonings.

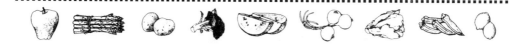

Fettuccine with Sautéed Onions, Meatless Bacon, and Green Peas in Lemon Sauce

SERVES 4 TO 6

Be sure to have plenty of good bread on hand for sopping up the light, luscious, lemon-flavored sauce. The meatless bacon I prefer is Fakin' Bacon by LightLife Foods.

¼ cup extra-virgin olive oil
3 medium sweet onions, finely chopped
4 large cloves garlic, finely chopped
1 6-ounce package meatless bacon, chopped (found in health food stores)
¼ cup finely chopped fresh Italian flat-leaf parsley
  Salt and pepper
1 cup water
1 cup dry white wine
1 bay leaf
2 teaspoons dried oregano
1 10-ounce box frozen tiny green peas
2 lemons, squeezed, about 6 tablespoons juice
3 eggs or equivalent egg substitute, lightly beaten
1 tablespoon arrowroot powder or cornstarch
1 pound fettuccine

Heat the olive oil in a large deep pot over medium heat. Add the onions, garlic, bacon, and parsley. Sprinkle with salt and pepper to taste. Cover and cook for 15 minutes, stirring occasionally, until the onions have released their juices. Stir in the water, wine, bay leaf, and oregano. Cover and cook at a medium boil for 30 minutes, stirring occasionally.

Meanwhile, cook the pasta according to package directions. Stir the green peas into the sauce. In a bowl, whisk together the lemon juice, salt and pepper to taste, and the eggs until well blended. Whisk in the arrowroot until well blended. Gradually pour this mixture into the sauce, stirring continuously as you pour. Cook, uncovered, stirring constantly for 2 minutes until the eggs are cooked. Remove the bay leaf. Stir in the cooked fettuccine and toss to coat with the sauce, using two spoons. Taste for seasonings.

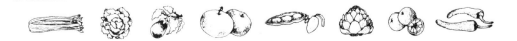

Farfalle with Peppers, Artichoke Hearts, and Capers in White Wine Sauce

SERVES 4 TO 6

This is my version of an old Sicilian favorite that my grandmother made during the summer, when the peppers were firm, plump, and fresh from Grandpa's garden.

- 4 tablespoons extra-virgin olive oil
- 6 large cloves garlic, coarsely chopped
- 1 medium onion, finely chopped
- 3 large red bell peppers, seeded and cut into ½-inch strips
  Salt and pepper
- 1 14-ounce can artichoke hearts, drained and sliced
- 3 tablespoons tiny capers, drained
- 1 teaspoon dried oregano
- 1 cup white wine
- 1 cup boiling water
- ½ cup finely chopped fresh Italian flat-leaf parsley
- 1 pound farfalle (bow tie) pasta

Heat the oil in a large deep skillet over medium heat. Add the garlic, onion, and peppers. Sprinkle with salt and pepper. Cover and cook for 30 minutes, stirring occasionally, until the peppers are crisp-tender. Stir in the artichoke hearts, capers, oregano, wine, water, and parsley. Cover and cook for 20 minutes, stirring occasionally, until the peppers are soft.

Meanwhile, cook the pasta according to package directions and drain. Taste the sauce for seasonings. Turn the cooked and drained pasta into a serving bowl. Pour the sauce over the pasta. Toss well to mix thoroughly, using two spoons.

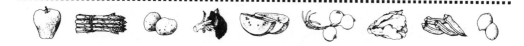

Fettuccine in Vodka Sauce with Garden Vegetables and "Sausage"

SERVES 4 TO 6

Although I love fettuccine noodles with this chunky sauce, if I'm feeling lazy I sometimes just serve it over big pieces of Italian bread to absorb the luscious juices. I use LightLife brand Italian meatless sausage links, found in health food stores and many supermarkets.

  2 tablespoons extra-virgin olive oil
  2 tablespoons soybean margarine (found in health food stores) or canola oil
  2 large cloves garlic, finely chopped
  1 large shallot, finely chopped
  2 medium onions, cut into ½-inch rings
  1 teaspoon crushed red pepper
  2 medium carrots, peeled and cut into ½-inch pieces
  ¼ pound green beans, trimmed and cut into 1-inch pieces (about 2 cups)
  ½ pound thin asparagus
  4 baby artichokes, quartered
    Salt and pepper
 12 shiitake mushrooms, stems discarded, caps cut in half
 12 large button mushrooms, cut in half
  3 medium potatoes, peeled, cut in half lengthwise, then into 1-inch slices
  1 35-ounce can Italian whole peeled tomatoes, with juice, squeezed with your hands to crush
  ¼ cup vodka
  1 12-ounce package meatless sausage, cut into 1-inch pieces
 12 large basil leaves, torn in half
  1 cup fresh or frozen green peas
  1 pound fettuccine

Remove the tough bottom (1 to 2 inches) of the asparagus and discard. Cut the remaining stalks into 1-inch pieces. Heat the olive oil and margarine in a large pot over low-medium heat. Add the garlic, shallot, onions, crushed red pepper, car-

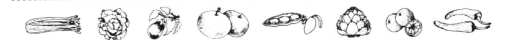

rots, green beans, asparagus, and artichokes. Sprinkle with salt and pepper to taste. Stir well to coat the vegetables with the oil and margarine. Cover and cook for 15 minutes, stirring occasionally, until the vegetables release some of their liquids. Add the mushrooms, potatoes, and tomatoes. Stir well to mix. Cover and raise the heat to medium. Bring to a boil (this should take about 10 minutes). Cook, covered, at a medium boil, stirring occasionally, for about 40 minutes, until the potatoes are soft and the artichokes are tender. Stir in the vodka, meatless sausage, basil, and green peas. Cover and continue cooking at a medium boil, stirring occasionally, for 20 minutes. Stir in salt and pepper to taste.

Meanwhile, cook the pasta according to package directions and drain. Turn the cooked and drained fettuccine into a serving bowl. Ladle about half of the sauce over the noodles. Toss to coat, using two spoons. Ladle the remaining sauce over the fettuccine.

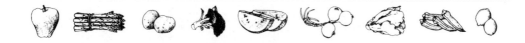

Linguine with Leeks, Red Onion, Carrots, Broccoli, and Asparagus

SERVES 4 TO 6

The carrots, asparagus, and broccoli florets in this flavorful dish are blanched before you add them to the sauce. You'll love the fresh taste of this chunky pasta meal.

- 3 medium carrots, peeled and cut into 1-inch julienne
- 1 pound asparagus, tough bottoms removed, cut into 1-inch pieces
- 1½ cups broccoli florets
- 3 tablespoons extra-virgin olive oil
- 6 large cloves garlic, minced
- 1 large leek, white part and 3 inches of green, finely chopped
- 2 medium onions, coarsely chopped
- 1 medium red (Bermuda) onion, finely chopped
  Salt and pepper
- ¼ cup finely chopped fresh Italian flat-leaf parsley
- 1 28-ounce can Italian peeled tomatoes, with juice, squeezed to crush with your hands
- ½ cup red Burgundy wine
- ¼ cup coarsely chopped fresh basil
- 1 tablespoon finely chopped fresh oregano or 1 teaspoon dried
- 1 teaspoon chopped fresh rosemary or ¼ teaspoon dried
- 1 bay leaf
- 1 pound linguine

Bring 2 quarts of lightly salted water to a boil in a covered pot over high heat. Add the carrots to the boiling water. Cover and cook for 1 minute. Add the asparagus stems. Cover and continue cooking for 3 minutes. Stir in the asparagus tips and the broccoli florets. Cover and continue cooking for 2 minutes. Set a colander in a large bowl. Carefully drain the vegetables, reserving the cooking water to use again to cook your linguine. Set the cooked vegetables aside.

Heat the olive oil in a wide skillet (3 to 4 inches deep) over low heat. Add the garlic, leeks, and yellow and red onions. Add salt and pepper to taste. Cover and cook over low heat for 20 minutes, stirring occasionally, until the garlic, leeks, and onions are softened and have released their liquids. Add the parsley, tomatoes, Burgundy, basil, oregano, rosemary, and bay leaf. Stir well to mix. Cover and continue cooking over low heat (it will come to a low-medium boil after 10 minutes or so) for about 25 minutes, stirring occasionally, until the sauce has reduced slightly. Stir in the cooked vegetables. Cover and continue cooking for 4 minutes, stirring occasionally. Taste for seasonings. Remove the bay leaf before serving.

Keep the sauce warm as you cook the linguine according to the package directions (remember to include the cooking water from blanching the vegetables). Drain and return the cooked linguine to the pot. Ladle half of the sauce over the linguine. Toss well to coat, using two spoons. Turn the linguine into a serving bowl. Top with remaining sauce.

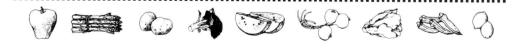

Linguine with Artichoke Hearts, Tomatoes, and Leeks

SERVES 6 TO 8

This chunky, Italian sauce is so flavorful, why not make a double batch and send a container over to a friend?

  4 tablespoons extra-virgin olive oil
  5 large cloves garlic, coarsely chopped
  2 medium sweet onions, coarsely chopped
  1 medium leek, white part and 3 inches of pale green, finely chopped
  2 teaspoons crushed red pepper
    Salt and pepper
¼ cup coarsely chopped fresh Italian flat-leaf parsley
  1 14-ounce can artichoke hearts, drained and cut into ¼-inch slices
  4 large ripe tomatoes, coarsely chopped (juices included)
  1 28-ounce can Italian whole peeled tomatoes, with juice, squeezed with your hands to crush
  3 tablespoons tomato paste
  1 cup water
¾ cup sweet vermouth
  1 bay leaf
10 large basil leaves
  1 teaspoon fennel seeds
1½ pounds linguine

Heat the olive oil in a large deep pot over medium heat. Add the garlic, onions, leeks, and crushed red pepper. Add salt and pepper to taste. Cover and cook for 10 minutes, stirring occasionally, until the leeks have released some of their liquids. Add the parsley, artichoke hearts, fresh tomatoes, canned tomatoes, tomato paste, water, vermouth, and bay leaf. Stir well to combine. Cover, raise the heat to medium high. Cook at a medium-high boil for 25 minutes, stirring occasionally. Stir in the basil leaves and fennel seeds. Continue cooking, uncovered, for 35 minutes, stirring occasionally, until the sauce has reduced by about a fourth. Remove the bay leaf.

Meanwhile, cook the pasta according to package directions. Taste the sauce for seasonings. Turn the cooked linguine into a serving bowl. Ladle half of the sauce over the linguine. Toss to coat the pasta. Ladle the remaining sauce over the top.

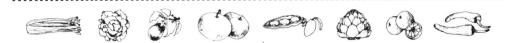

Farfalle with Tomatoes and Swiss Chard

SERVES 4 TO 6

Nella Alberta, a marvelous Sicilian cook who now lives in Boston, generously shared this delicious recipe with her sister, my good friend Tina, who passed it on to me. It's been a big hit at my house. Swiss chard is rich in vitamins A and C and is available year-round. Look for small tender leaves when you choose your chard.

- 4 tablespoons extra-virgin olive
- 6 large cloves garlic, coarsely chopped
- 1 large leek, white part and 5 inches of pale green, coarsely chopped
- 4 large ripe tomatoes, coarsely chopped, including juices
- 2 teaspoons dried oregano
  Salt and pepper
- 1 pound farfalle pasta (bow ties)
- 1 large bunch Swiss chard, tough ribs discarded, washed well and coarsely chopped

Heat the olive oil in a large deep sauté pan over medium heat. Add the garlic and leek. Cook for 5 minutes, stirring occasionally, until the leeks have released some of their liquids. Stir in the tomatoes and oregano. Sprinkle with salt and pepper to taste. Cover and cook for 25 minutes, stirring occasionally, until the tomatoes are soft and have broken up. Taste for seasonings.

Meanwhile, bring a large pot of water to a boil over high heat. Add the pasta and the Swiss chard. Sprinkle with salt and pepper. Cook, stirring occasionally, until the pasta is just tender. Drain the pasta and the Swiss chard. After the tomatoes have cooked, add the pasta and the Swiss chard to the sauce. Stir well to combine. Cover and cook for 3 minutes, stirring occasionally, until the flavors are well blended. Taste for seasonings. Serve with additional pepper on top if you want.

Orzo with Oven-Roasted Vegetables

SERVES 6 TO 8

This delicious dish was inspired by my neighbor Alice Samaras. She is a marvelous cook who draws upon her Greek/Turkish heritage for inspiration. Rice-shaped orzo pasta is very popular in Greece, and I find that it makes a lovely change both from regular pasta and rice!

1 medium eggplant (about 1 pound), unpeeled and cut into ½-inch pieces
1 medium cucumber, peeled, seeded, and cut into 1-inch pieces
1 medium zucchini (about 1 pound), cut into 1-inch pieces
1 medium red (Bermuda) onion, peeled and cut into 1-inch pieces
1 medium sweet onion, peeled and cut into 1-inch pieces
2 medium potatoes, peeled and cut into ½-inch pieces
2 medium tomatoes, cut into 1-inch pieces
4 large cloves garlic, coarsely chopped
1 14-ounce can artichoke hearts, coarsely chopped
¼ cup extra-virgin olive oil
¼ cup water
  Salt and pepper
2 teaspoons dried oregano
¼ cup currants
1 to 2 lemons, squeezed, about ¼ cup juice
1 tablespoon freshly grated orange zest
1 pound orzo
8 ounces dill Havarti cheese, cut into ½-inch cubes

Preheat the oven to 400 degrees. Place the eggplant, cucumber, zucchini, onions, potatoes, tomatoes, garlic, and artichoke hearts in a large mixing bowl. Toss together to mix. Pour the olive oil and the water over the top and stir to mix well, using two spoons or your hands. Add the salt and pepper to taste and the oregano. Toss together to mix well. Spray a large deep casserole pan with olive oil spray or other cooking oil spray to coat evenly. Turn the vegetables into the

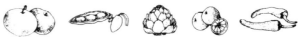

prepared pan, using a spatula to scrape out all of the juices. Cover the pan tightly with foil. Bake on the lower shelf of the oven for 30 minutes.

Remove the pan from the oven and carefully remove the foil. Stir the vegetables to mix. Cover and continue baking for another 15 minutes until the eggplant is soft when tested with a fork. Remove the pan from the oven and stir in the currants, lemon juice, and orange zest. Mix well.

Meanwhile, cook the orzo pasta according to package directions. Drain well then return it to the pot. When the roasted vegetables are ready, add them to the cooked orzo and toss to mix together. Stir in the Havarti cheese. Stir for about 2 minutes until the cheese melts. Taste for seasonings. Serve immediately.

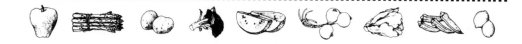

Noodles and Mushrooms in Creamy Sherry Sauce

SERVES 4

I can't think of many dishes more luscious than pappardelle pasta in a rich, creamy sauce with shiitake, cremini, and button mushrooms. And I can't think of any more delicious way to enjoy the many benefits of eating soy products.

- 3 tablespoons soybean margarine (found in health food stores) or canola oil
- 2 large shallots, minced
- 1 pound assorted shiitake, cremini, and button mushrooms, stems discarded, cut into ¼-inch slices
- 1 pound pappardelle or fettuccine
- 3 tablespoons flour
- ¼ cup sweet sherry
- 3 cups soy milk
- ⅛ teaspoon nutmeg
- ⅛ teaspoon ground red pepper (cayenne)
  Salt and pepper

Melt the soy margarine or heat the oil in a large deep sauté pan over medium heat. Add the shallots. Cover and cook for 5 minutes, stirring occasionally, until softened. Add the mushrooms. Stir well to coat with the melted margarine or oil. Cover and cook for about 25 minutes, stirring occasionally, until the mushrooms are tender.

Meanwhile, cook the pasta according to package directions while you finish the sauce: Sprinkle the flour evenly over the mushrooms. Stir well to combine. Cook, uncovered, stirring and scraping the pan constantly, using a wooden spoon, for about 3 minutes. Gradually add the sherry and soy milk, stirring continuously. Stir in the nutmeg, cayenne, and salt and pepper to taste. Cook for about 5 minutes, stirring frequently, until the mixture thickens slightly. Add the cooked, drained pappardelle to the sauté pan and toss to coat the pasta evenly, using two spoons. Taste for seasonings. Serve immediately.

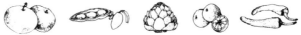

Pappardelle with Shiitake, Cremini, and Button Mushroom Sauce

SERVES 4 TO 6

Pappardelle are tender, wide ribbons of pasta, traditionally served with fragrant wild mushroom sauces. Unfortunately, I can't always find real pappardelle except in an Italian gourmet store. Wide fettuccine noodles are a fine second choice. Either way, this sauce is a winner.

1 pound pappardelle or fettuccine
⅓ cup plus 1 teaspoon extra-virgin olive oil
1 medium leek, white part and 4 inches of green, finely chopped
4 large cloves garlic, coarsely chopped
1½ pounds assorted mushrooms, (shiitake, cremini, and button), stems discarded, cut into ¼-inch slices
2 tablespoons steak sauce
¼ cup sweet vermouth
Salt and pepper

Cook the pasta according to package directions. Reserve ⅓ cup of cooking water. Drain the pasta. Rinse under cold water. Drain. Toss with 1 teaspoon of the olive oil. Set aside. In a large skillet, heat ⅓ cup olive oil over a low-medium heat. Add the leeks and the garlic. Cover and cook for 5 minutes, stirring occasionally, until the leeks are softened. Add the sliced mushrooms, steak sauce, and vermouth. Sprinkle with salt and pepper to taste. Stir to mix. Cover and continue cooking for 10 minutes, stirring occasionally. Stir in the reserved ⅓ cup of pasta cooking liquid. Raise heat to medium. Cover and continue cooking for 5 to 7 minutes at a low-medium boil, stirring occasionally, until the mushrooms are tender. Turn the cooked pasta into the sauce. Gently toss together, using two spoons, until the pasta is well coated with the sauce. Cover and continue cooking for 3 minutes, gently stirring occasionally, until heated through. Taste for seasonings.

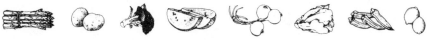

Pappardelle with Vegetable Cacciatore

SERVES 8

This chunky, well-spiced, luscious sauce is one of my favorite Italian sauces, especially when served over wide pappardelle pasta. Unfortunately, pappardelle are not readily available at the local supermarkets, so I settle for wide egg noodles. But when I do come across pappardelle, those beautiful, long ribbons of tender pasta, I buy several packages and strongly recommend that you do the same.

¼ cup plus 2 tablespoons extra-virgin olive oil
2 medium sweet onions, cut into ½-inch ribs
1 large red (Bermuda) onion, cut into ½-inch ribs
8 large cloves garlic, coarsely chopped
4 large carrots, peeled and cut on the diagonal into ½-inch pieces
6 ribs celery with leaves, cut into 1-inch pieces
   Salt and pepper
2 medium potatoes, peeled and cut into 3-inch spears
½ pound mixed portobello, cremini, and shiitake mushrooms, sliced (discard the stems of the shiitakes)
7 large ripe tomatoes, coarsely chopped (include the juices)
1 6-ounce can tomato paste
½ cup finely chopped fresh Italian flat-leaf parsley
1 cup red wine
1 tablespoon dried thyme
1 teaspoon dried sage
1 teaspoon dried oregano leaves
1 pinch ground red pepper (cayenne)
1 bay leaf
1 pound extra-firm tofu, drained and cut into ½-inch cubes
1 pound pappardelle or wide egg noodles

Heat the oil in a large deep skillet over low-medium heat. Add the onions, garlic, carrots, and celery. Sprinkle with salt and pepper. Cover and cook for 15

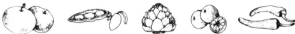

minutes, stirring occasionally, until the onions are wilted. Add the potatoes and the mushrooms. Sprinkle lightly with salt. Cover and continue cooking for 10 minutes, stirring occasionally, until the mushrooms have released some of their liquid.

Add the tomatoes, tomato paste, parsley, wine, thyme, sage, oregano, cayenne, and bay leaf. Sprinkle generously with salt and pepper. Stir to combine. Raise the heat to medium. Cover and cook at a medium boil for about 50 minutes, stirring frequently (push the potatoes to the bottom of the pot so they are always covered by sauce, in order to fully cook them) until the sauce is rich and slightly reduced. Gently stir in the tofu, mixing carefully, trying to keep the cubes of tofu intact. Taste for seasonings. Remove the bay leaf. Keep the sauce warm while you cook the pasta according to package directions. Drain the pasta. Turn into a serving bowl. Ladle about a fourth of the sauce over the noodles. Toss gently but thoroughly using two spoons. Top with a ladle or two of additional sauce. Ladle extra sauce into a bowl for passing. Serve with good bread for sopping up extra sauce.

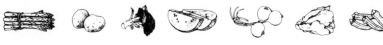

Penne with Roasted Potatoes, Onions, and Green Peas in Lemon-Wine Sauce

SERVES 4 TO 6

This delicious pasta is truly a complete meal, providing an abundance of vegetables: The potatoes are roasted with the onions and the green peas are tossed with a little olive oil and herbs. Then you sauté mushrooms and shallots in extra-virgin olive oil, with white wine and fresh lemon juice added toward the end. All that remains is to add some good Italian bread and perhaps a simple tossed salad to make a lovely dinner.

- 6 large white potatoes
- 2 large sweet onions (preferably Vidalia), cut in half, then sliced into ½-inch ribs
- 2 cloves garlic, minced
- 6 tablespoons extra-virgin olive oil
- 1 tablespoon fresh rosemary
- 1 teaspoon paprika
  Salt and pepper
- 1 10-ounce package frozen green peas
- 1 pound penne pasta
- 2 large shallots, thinly sliced
- 6 large or 8 medium shiitake mushrooms, stems discarded, cut into ¼-inch slices
- 1 tablespoon chopped fresh thyme or 1 teaspoon dried
- 2 lemons, squeezed, about 6 tablespoons juice
- ½ cup white wine

Preheat oven to 400 degrees. Peel the potatoes. Cut into ½-inch slices, placing the potatoes in a bowl of cold water (to cover them) to prevent discoloration as you cut the potatoes. Drain the potatoes well. Turn into a bowl. Add the onions and garlic. Drizzle with 3 tablespoons of the olive oil. Sprinkle with the rose-

     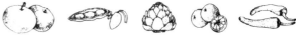

mary, paprika, and salt and pepper to taste. Spray a large rectangular baking dish with nonstick cooking spray. Turn the potato mixture into the prepared baking dish. Spread evenly, using a spoon. Bake for about 45 minutes, turning occasionally, until the potatoes are tender and golden brown. Stir in the peas. Remove from the oven. Set aside.

Put the water on to boil for the pasta, and cook it according to the package directions while you finish the sauce, reserving ¼ cup of the cooking liquid before draining. Heat the remaining 3 tablespoons of olive oil in a large skillet over low-medium heat. Add the shallots and mushrooms. Sprinkle with salt and pepper to taste and the thyme. Stir to combine. Cook for 5 minutes, stirring occasionally, until the mushrooms are barely tender. Add the lemon juice, wine, and the reserved ¼ cup of cooking liquid from the pasta. Raise the heat to medium-high. Bring to a boil. Cook at a medium boil for 5 minutes, stirring frequently. Taste for seasonings. Remove from the heat. In a large bowl, combine the cooked pasta, the potato mixture, all the pan juices, and the sautéed mushrooms (use a rubber spatula to scrape the skillet). Toss well to mix the ingredients. Taste for seasonings. Serve immediately.

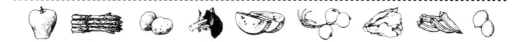

Penne with San Marzano Tomatoes, Shiitake Mushrooms, Leeks, and Vermouth

MAKES ABOUT 3 QUARTS, ENOUGH FOR 3 POUNDS OF PASTA

San Marzano tomatoes are grown only in San Marzano, just as our sweet Vidalia onions are grown only in Vidalia, Georgia. Although I enjoy all of the tomatoes grown and packed in Italy, these are special. They are more flavorful than any others, silky soft in texture, and absolutely worth the trouble you may have in locating them. Ask for San Marzano tomatoes (not San Marzano-style) at either an Italian import store or at your supermarket. Although you can certainly substitute any Italian tomatoes, I promise you that the tomatoes from San Marzano will make the best sauce you ever tasted.

¼ cup extra-virgin olive oil
4 large cloves garlic, chopped
2 large leeks, white part and 3 inches of green, finely chopped
1 large red (Bermuda) onion, finely chopped
½ pound shiitake mushrooms, stems discarded, cut into thin strips
½ cup dry vermouth
   Salt and pepper
2 28-ounce cans Italian peeled tomatoes, with juice, squeezed with your hands to crush
1 6-ounce can tomato paste
2 cups water
½ cup chopped fresh basil
¼ cup finely chopped fresh Italian flat-leaf parsley
1 pound penne pasta

Heat the oil in large deep skillet over low heat. Add the garlic, leeks, and red onion. Cover and cook for 20 minutes, stirring occasionally, until the onions and leeks are softened. Add the mushrooms and vermouth. Add salt and pepper to taste. Stir well to mix. Cover and continue cooking for 5 minutes, stirring occa-

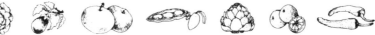

sionally. Add the tomatoes, tomato paste, water, basil, and parsley. Stir well to mix. Cover and raise the heat to medium. Bring the sauce to a boil, then reduce the heat to low-medium. Continue cooking, covered, at a low to medium boil for about 1 hour, stirring occasionally, until the sauce is reduced by about a third.

Put the water on to boil for your pasta, and cook it according to the package directions while you finish the sauce. When the pasta is cooked, drain it and turn it into a serving bowl. Taste the sauce (a piece of Italian bread is great for tasting) to see if you need to add additional salt and pepper. Add about 2 cups of the sauce to your bowl of pasta. Toss well to coat. Top with an additional 2 cups of sauce.

NOTE: Freeze (or share) the remaining sauce in 2 separate containers and eat it within a month. Use it on pasta, over polenta, or on bread for pizzas.

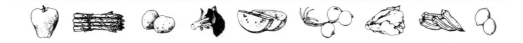

Penne with Tofu Sausage, Mushrooms, Black Olives, and Pepperoncini in Marsala Wine Sauce

SERVES 4 to 6

The contrast between the sweetness of the marsala wine and the saltiness of the olives is picked up by the pickled flavor of the pepperoncini in this traditional southern Italian dish. The meatless (tofu) sausage I prefer is LightLife brand Italian Lean Links, found in health food stores.

- 8 ounces assorted mushrooms (cremini, oyster, and shiitake), stems discarded, cut into ¼-inch slices
- 1 tablespoons extra-virgin olive oil
- 2 tablespoons soybean margarine (found in health food stores) or canola oil
- 2 shallots, minced
- 2 large cloves garlic, minced
- 1 large sweet onion, chopped
- 1 12-ounce package of meatless (tofu) sausage, cut into 1-inch pieces
- 1 pound penne pasta
- 1 6-ounce can medium-size pitted black olives, drained
- 15 pepperoncini peppers (sold in jars in the Italian section of supermarkets)
- 2 cups marsala wine
  Salt and pepper
- ½ teaspoon arrowroot or cornstarch

Heat the olive oil and margarine in a large sauté pan over medium heat. Add the shallots, garlic, onion, and mushrooms. Cover and cook for 5 minutes, stirring occasionally. Add the tofu sausage and continue cooking, uncovered, for 15 minutes, stirring occasionally. Put the water on to boil for your pasta, and cook it according to the package directions while you finish the sauce. When the pasta is cooked, drain it and turn it into a serving bowl. To the sauce in the skillet, add the olives, pepperoncini peppers, and 1 cup of the marasala. Sprinkle with salt and pepper to taste. Raise heat to medium high and bring to a boil. Cook at a medium boil for 12 minutes, stirring occasionally.

In a separate cup, whisk together the remaining cup of marsala and the arrow-root. Add to the skillet and reduce the heat to low. Continue cooking for 5 minutes, stirring frequently, until the sauce thickens slightly. Add the cooked pasta to the skillet. Toss well to mix. Taste for seasonings.

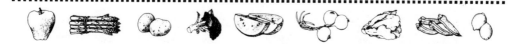

Rigatoni with Tomatoes, Mushrooms, Pernod, and Goat Cheese

MAKES 8 TO 12 SERVINGS

The first time that I tasted Pernod was many years ago in a delightful little Italian restaurant in an obscure part of New Haven. The restaurant has long since closed, and while I don't recall the name or even the exact location of the restaurant, I clearly remember the marvelous dish that my dear friend Phyllis and I shared. It was an angel hair pasta dish with shrimp, in a wonderful tomato sauce with an unusual flavor I couldn't identify. The waiter told me that it was Pernod, a licorice-flavored liqueur that you can buy at any liquor store. Although I haven't eaten shrimp for many years, I never did get that wonderful dish out of my mind. Here is my version, made with creamy white oyster mushrooms and woodsy-flavored shiitake mushrooms.

½ cup extra-virgin olive oil
8 large cloves garlic, finely chopped
1 medium leek, white part and 3 inches of green, finely chopped
12 medium (about ⅓ pound) shiitake mushrooms, stems discarded, caps cut into ¼-inch slices
12 medium (about ¼ pound) oyster mushrooms, cut into ¼-inch slices
¼ cup chopped fresh Italian flat-leaf parsley
1 small hot red cherry pepper, finely chopped (wash your hands immediately after handling hot peppers)
 Salt and pepper
½ cup Pernod
2 teaspoons fennel seeds
2 28-ounce cans Italian whole peeled tomatoes in juice, squeezed with your hands to crush
1 6-ounce can tomato paste
2 cups water
1 bay leaf

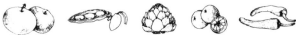

⅛ teaspoon crushed red pepper
 2 pounds rigatoni
12 large basil leaves
 1 cup frozen petite green peas
 2 ounces goat cheese

Heat the oil in a large deep skillet over low-medium heat. Add the garlic, leek, mushrooms, parsley, and cherry pepper. Sprinkle with salt and pepper to taste. Cook for 10 minutes, stirring occasionally, until the leeks are softened. Stir in the Pernod and the fennel seeds. Cook for 5 minutes, stirring occasionally. Add the tomatoes, tomato paste, water, bay leaf, and crushed red pepper. Stir well to combine. Raise the heat to medium. Bring to a low-medium boil, then lower the heat to low-medium. Cook, uncovered, at a low-medium boil for 40 minutes, stirring occasionally.

Put the water on to boil for your pasta, and cook it according to the package directions while you finish the sauce. Stir the basil leaves and the green peas into the sauce. Continue cooking for 10 minutes, stirring occasionally. Stir in the goat cheese. Cook for 5 minutes, stirring frequently, until the cheese is melted into the sauce. Remove the bay leaf. Taste for seasonings.

After draining the pasta briefly, turn it into a serving bowl. Add about a fourth of the sauce. Toss to coat the pasta. Spoon about half of the remaining sauce over the pasta. Grind black pepper over the top. Spoon remaining sauce into a bowl to pass at the table. Serve immediately.

Rigatoni with Green Beans and Tomatoes

SERVES 4 TO 6

My mom has always been a big fan of green beans and she serves them in a variety of ways. They appear in salads, soups, stews, and in this flavorful, traditional southern Italian sauce.

¼ cup extra-virgin olive oil
2 medium sweet onions, finely chopped
4 large cloves garlic, finely chopped
1 pound green beans, trimmed and cut into 1-inch pieces (about 2½ cups)
  Salt and pepper
2 large ripe tomatoes, coarsely chopped
1 35-ounce can Italian whole peeled tomatoes, with juice, squeezed with your hands to crush
3 tablespoons tomato paste
1 cup water
1 teaspoon dried oregano
10 large basil leaves
1 bay leaf
¼ cup coarsely chopped fresh Italian flat-leaf parsley
1 pound rigatoni pasta
  Freshly grated Parmesan cheese (optional)

Heat the olive oil in a large deep pot over medium heat. Add the onions, garlic, and green beans. Sprinkle with salt and pepper. Cover and cook for 15 minutes, stirring occasionally, until the onions release their juices. Add the ripe tomatoes, canned tomatoes, tomato paste, water, oregano, basil, bay leaf, and parsley. Cover and bring to a medium boil, stirring occasionally. This should take about 10 minutes. Cook, covered, at a medium boil for about 45 minutes more, stirring occasionally until the green beans are tender and the sauce has reduced slightly. Taste for seasonings. Remove the bay leaf.

Cover the sauce and keep warm while you cook the pasta according to package directions. Drain the pasta and turn it into the sauce. Stir to coat the pasta with the sauce until it is heated through. Top with grated Parmesan cheese and freshly ground black pepper, if desired.

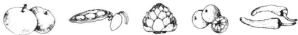

Pasta Puttanesca

SERVES 4 TO 6

This spicy, richly flavored sauce is perfect over linguine noodles but is also great with spaghetti or capellini. Serve it with sautéed Italian-style greens (escarole, broccoli rabe, or dandelion greens) and Roasted Bell Peppers with Capers, Olives, and Oregano (page 78) for a delightful Italian supper. Don't forget the Italian bread.

- 3 tablespoons extra-virgin olive oil
- 6 cloves garlic, minced
- 1 medium sweet onion (preferably Vidalia), chopped
- ¼ cup oil-cured olives, pitted
- 6 pepperoncini peppers (found in jars at the supermarket)
- 2 tablespoons tiny capers, drained
- ¼ cup pimiento-stuffed Spanish olives
- 1 tablespoon chopped hot cherry peppers (wash your hands immediately after handling hot peppers)
- ½ cup chopped fresh Italian flat-leaf parsley
- 1 28-ounce can Italian peeled tomatoes (San Marzano, if available), with juice
- ½ cup water
- ½ teaspoon dried oregano
- ⅛ teaspoon ground red pepper (cayenne)
  Salt and pepper
- 1 pound linguine

Heat the oil in a large deep skillet over low heat. Add the garlic and onion. Cover and cook for 4 minutes, stirring occasionally, until the garlic and onions are softened but not browned. Add the oil-cured olives, pepperoncini peppers, capers, Spanish olives, hot peppers, and parsley. Cover and cook for 5 minutes, stirring occasionally. Add the tomatoes, water, oregano, and cayenne. Sprinkle lightly with salt (remember, the olives and capers are salty) and pepper to taste. Cover. The sauce will gradually come to a boil. Cook, covered, over low heat for about 45 minutes, stirring occasionally, until the sauce reduces and thickens slightly. Taste for seasonings.

Meanwhile, put the water on to boil for your pasta, and cook it according to the package directions while you finish the sauce. When the pasta is cooked, drain it and return it to the pot. Ladle one third of the sauce over the top. Toss well to mix, using two spoons. Turn into a serving bowl. Top with the remaining sauce.

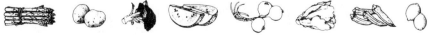

Rigatoni with "Sausages," Mushrooms, and Italian-Style Tofu

SERVES 6

Since I've discovered Italian-style tofu sausages, there is nothing to stop me from enjoying richly flavored dishes from my meat-eating days. Everyone I've introduced them to appreciates these delicious, guilt-free sausages. I use LightLife brand Italian links, found in health food stores.

- 1 10½-ounce package extra-firm lite tofu (found in health food stores)
- 2 tablespoons flour
- 2 teaspoons dried oregano
- 1 teaspoon garlic powder
- 1 teaspoon onion powder
  Salt and pepper
- ¼ cup extra-virgin olive oil
- 1 11-ounce package meatless Italian-style sausages, cut into ¼-inch pieces while partially frozen
- 3 large green bell peppers, seeded and cut into ½-inch ribs
- 1 pound mixed button and cremini mushrooms, cut into ¼-inch slices
- 1 cup red wine vinegar
- 1 cup tap water
- 10 large fresh basil leaves
- 1 bay leaf
- 1 cup boiling water
- ¼ teaspoon ground red pepper (cayenne)
- 1 pound rigatoni
  Freshly grated Romano or Asiago cheese (optional)

Drain the tofu in a colander for 20 minutes, then cut the block into ½-inch cubes. Line a cookie sheet with a double layer of paper towels. Arrange the tofu cubes in a single layer on the paper towels to dry. Cover with a double layer of

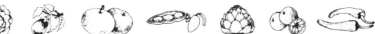

paper towels. Press down gently to dry the tofu cubes. In a shallow bowl, combine the flour, oregano, garlic powder, onion powder, and salt and pepper to taste. Whisk to combine. Add the tofu cubes to the flour mixture, a few at a time, tossing well to coat evenly. Lift them out, using your hands, shaking off the excess. Transfer to a plate. Repeat, coating all of the tofu cubes.

Heat the olive oil in a large deep skillet over medium heat. Add the tofu cubes and the sausages. Cook for about 5 minutes, stirring occasionally, and scraping the bottom of the pan, using a wooden spoon, until the sausages are golden brown. Add the peppers, mushrooms, vinegar, tap water, basil, and bay leaf. Sprinkle with salt and pepper to taste. Stir well to combine. Cover and cook for about 30 minutes (it will come to a medium boil after about 15 minutes), stirring occasionally, until the peppers are crisp-tender. Stir in the boiling water and the cayenne. Cover and continue cooking for 10 minutes, stirring occasionally. Remove the bay leaf.

Meanwhile, cook the pasta according to package directions and drain. Stir the cooked pasta into the sauce. Taste for seasonings. Top with freshly grated Asiago or Romano cheese, if desired.

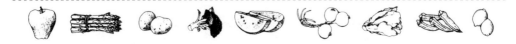

Rigatoni with Mushrooms in a Creamy Whisky Sauce

SERVES 4 TO 6

This outstanding sauce combines the rich, woodsy flavors of cremini, shiitake, oyster, and portobello mushrooms with the delicate smoothness of a cream sauce. This fabulous sauce is cholesterol-free and even has the added goodness of soy.

3 tablespoons soybean margarine (found in health food stores) or canola oil
4 large shallots, finely chopped
1 pound assorted mushrooms (cremini, shiitake, oyster, and portobello), stems discarded, cut into ¼-inch slices
Salt and pepper
¼ cup Scotch whisky
½ cup coarsely chopped fresh basil
4 cups soy milk
1 pound rigatoni
3 tablespoons arrowroot powder or cornstarch

Melt margarine in a large deep skillet over low heat. Add the shallots, mushrooms, and salt and pepper to taste. Stir to mix. Cover and cook for 15 minutes, stirring occasionally, until the mushrooms are just softened and have released their liquids. Add the Scotch and the basil. Cover and continue cooking for 5 minutes, stirring occasionally. Stir in 3 cups of the soy milk. Cover and continue cooking for 30 minutes, stirring occasionally as it cooks (it will reach a boil after about 15 minutes) at a low-medium boil.

Put the water on to boil for your pasta, and cook it according to the package directions while you finish the sauce. In a bowl, whisk together the remaining 1 cup of soy milk with the arrowroot powder until smooth. Remove the sauce from the heat. Stir in the arrowroot mixture all at once. Return to the heat. Stir continuously for 1 minute. It will thicken right away. Add the cooked pasta to the sauce. Stir together over low heat until heated through. Taste for seasonings.

Sesame Noodles

SERVES 4

*At **Claire's** and at home, we've always served this wonderful, richly flavored, Chinese pasta salad cold. Hot or cold, I love its distinctive peanut butter and hot chili pepper flavor. Serve it for dinner with Broccoli with Garlic Chips (page 87) and Sautéed Green Beans, Carrots, and Shiitake Mushrooms (page 85). Take any leftovers along for lunch the next day. Just toss it to mix the noodles and dressing before you eat it.*

- ½ pound linguine
- 2 teaspoons sesame oil
- 2 large cloves garlic, minced
- 2 teaspoons hot chili paste or crushed red pepper
- ¾ cup creamy peanut butter
- ¼ cup rice vinegar
- ½ cup soy sauce
- ¾ cup water
- 2 tablespoons honey
- Salt and pepper
- 1 medium cucumber, peeled, seeded, cut in half lengthwise, then into ¼-inch slices
- 1 tablespoon sesame seeds

Cook the linguine according to package directions. Drain. Turn into a large bowl. Drizzle 1 teaspoon of the sesame oil evenly over the noodles. Toss well to coat, using two spoons. Heat the remaining 1 teaspoon of sesame oil in a pot over low-medium heat. Add the garlic and the hot chili paste. Cook for 5 minutes, stirring frequently, until the garlic is softened but not browned. Stir in the peanut butter, rice vinegar, ¼ cup of the soy sauce, the water, honey, and salt and pepper to taste. Stir to mix thoroughly. Cook for 3 minutes stirring frequently, until the mixture has become smooth and creamy. Taste for seasonings.

Pour the sauce over the noodles. Toss thoroughly using two spoons to coat the noodles evenly. Turn the noodles into a large, serving bowl. Scatter the cucumber slices and the sesame seeds evenly over the noodles. Drizzle the remaining ¼ cup of soy sauce evenly over the noodles. Serve immediately or refrigerate and serve chilled. Toss again just before serving to coat the noodles with the dressing.

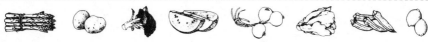

Tortellini in Creamy Tomato Sauce with Artichoke Hearts

SERVES 4 TO 6

This sauce is so delicious that you can enjoy it over any pasta, but it really is perfect over tortellini. Of course, you can use cheese tortellini, but do visit your health food store and try some tofu tortellini because it tastes great with this sauce.

3 tablespoons soybean margarine (found in health food stores) or canola oil
1 medium leek, white part and 4 inches of pale green, finely chopped
2 large cloves garlic, finely chopped
¼ cup finely chopped fresh Italian flat-leaf parsley
   Salt and pepper
1 28-ounce can Italian peeled tomatoes, with juice, squeezed with your hands to crush
¼ cup tomato paste
1 cup water
⅓ cup coarsely chopped fresh basil (chop it just before you add it to the sauce)
1 14-ounce can artichoke hearts, drained and sliced
¼ teaspoon ground red pepper (cayenne)
1 pound tofu or cheese tortellini
1 cup soy milk (found in most supermarkets and in health food stores)

Melt the margarine or heat the oil in a large pot over medium heat. Add the leeks, garlic, and parsley. Sprinkle with salt and pepper to taste. Cover and cook for 10 minutes, stirring occasionally, until the leeks are softened and have released their liquids. Add the tomatoes, tomato paste, and water. Stir well to mix. Cover and bring to a boil over medium heat. This should take about 10 minutes. Cook, covered, at a medium to rapid boil for 25 minutes more, stirring occasionally. Stir in the basil, artichoke hearts, and cayenne.

Meanwhile, cook the pasta according to package directions while you finish the sauce. Gradually add the soy milk into the sauce, stirring continuously as you pour. Stir well to mix. Add salt and pepper to taste. Continue cooking, uncovered, at a medium boil, stirring frequently for 5 minutes. Add the cooked and drained tortellini to the sauce. Stir well to mix. Cook, uncovered, for 5 minutes, stirring frequently until the sauce thickens slightly. Taste for seasonings.

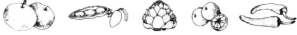

Linguine with Extra-Virgin Olive Oil, Garlic, and Walnuts

SERVES 4 TO 6

On some occasions my mom made a delicious yet simple dish of linguine tossed with sautéed garlic in olive oil for dinner on Fridays (like most Italian Catholics, we abstained from eating meat on Friday). I was about to make this flavorful dish one night when my friend Louise Povinelli told me about her mom's version. It is similar to my mom's but has chopped walnuts and finely grated fresh lemon zest—the flavor is wonderful.

  1 **pound linguine**
  ½ **cup extra-virgin olive oil**
 12 **large cloves garlic, thinly sliced**
  1 **teaspoon crushed red pepper**
  ¼ **cup finely chopped fresh Italian flat-leaf parsley**
  ¼ **cup chopped walnuts**
    Salt and pepper
  1 **tablespoon freshly grated lemon zest**
    Freshly grated Parmesan cheese (optional)

Cook the pasta according to package directions, reserving ½ cup of cooking liquid before draining. Meanwhile, heat the olive oil in a large skillet over low-medium heat. Add the garlic and crushed red pepper. Cook for 5 minutes, stirring occasionally, until the garlic is softened and golden brown. Add the parsley, reserved cooking liquid from the pasta, and walnuts. Continue cooking for 5 minutes, stirring occasionally. Sprinkle with salt and pepper. Add the cooked linguine to the skillet. Mix well, using tongs to turn the pasta to coat evenly. Sprinkle with the lemon zest. Toss again. Taste for seasonings. Turn into a serving bowl. Serve immediately. Pass the grated Parmesan cheese, if using.

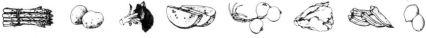

Ziti with Escarole, Potatoes, and Sun-Dried Tomatoes

SERVES 6

Escarole is a member of the endive family, but it looks more like a leafy head of lettuce. This is a popular green in the Italian community and we use it in many soups, sautéed as a side dish, and basically in any dish that calls for some delicious, healthy greens. Roasted Bell Peppers with Capers, Olives, and Oregano (page 78) round out this meal nicely. Serve the pasta in bowls, grate a little Asiago cheese over the top, and have plenty of hard-crusted Italian bread ready for sopping up every wonderful drop.

  4 tablespoons extra-virgin olive oil
  6 large cloves garlic, coarsely chopped
  1 medium onion, finely chopped
  ¼ cup finely chopped fresh Italian flat-leaf parsley
  1 teaspoon crushed red pepper
  2 large heads escarole, leaves cut in half lengthwise
  ¼ cup thinly sliced, sun-dried tomatoes, drained if oil-packed
  3 medium potatoes, peeled, sliced into ¼-inch rounds
10 calamata olives, pitted and cut in half
  1 tablespoon tiny capers, drained
  4 cups water
   Salt and pepper
  1 pound ziti

Heat the olive oil in a large pot over medium heat. Add the garlic, onion, parsley, and crushed red pepper. Cover and cook for 5 minutes, stirring occasionally, until the onions are softened but not brown. Add the escarole. Cover and cook for 20 minutes, stirring occasionally, until the leaves are crisp-tender.

Scatter the slices of tomatoes evenly over the escarole. Arrange the potatoes over the tomatoes. Scatter the olives and capers over the potatoes. Pour the water over the potatoes. Sprinkle lightly with salt and pepper. Cover and bring to a boil over medium heat. This should take about 15 minutes. Cook, covered, at a

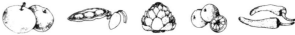

medium-high boil for about 35 minutes, stirring occasionally, until the potatoes are soft and falling apart (this will thicken the broth) and the escarole is tender. Taste for seasonings.

Meanwhile, cook the pasta according to package directions. Turn the cooked (and drained) ziti into the pot of cooked escarole and potatoes. Stir well to mix. Cover and cook for 5 minutes, stirring frequently. Taste for seasonings. Serve immediately.

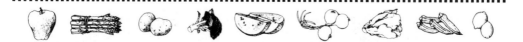

Ziti with Fava Beans and Dandelion Greens

SERVES 8

This is one of the most delicious combinations I have ever eaten (and I have cooked and eaten a lot in my life!). I first noticed fava beans in an Italian market in Florida, where you can buy dried beans from huge barrels set on the floor. Fava beans are large, flat, tan beans that resemble jumbo lima beans. When I asked the cashier about how to prepare these beans, she suggested that I cook them with Swiss chard. Well on this particular February day the dandelion greens were piled high and were a particularly beautiful dark green. I couldn't resist. I serve this dish with Fresh Corn Polenta with Tomatoes and Basil Ricotta (page 115) and Orange-Maple Carrots (page 92). Note: If you are picking your own dandelion greens, be it in the wild or from your own yard, please use caution. Pesticides and fertilizers may have been used and can be hazardous to your health.

  1 pound fava beans (2 cups), picked over and soaked overnight in the refrigerator, then drained
14 cloves garlic, finely chopped, divided
¼ plus ⅓ cup extra-virgin olive oil
¼ cup coarsely chopped fresh Italian flat-leaf parsley
  2 large leeks, white part and 3 inches of green, coarsely chopped
  2 large bunches dandelion greens, washed well and chopped into 2-inch pieces (about 2 pounds)
  6 medium ripe tomatoes, chopped (include juices)
1½ teaspoons crushed red pepper
  1 teaspoon dried oregano
    Salt and pepper
  1 pound ziti pasta

Put the soaked fava beans and 3 quarts of water into an 8-quart pot. Cover and bring to a boil over high heat. Stir in 8 cloves chopped garlic, ¼ cup of the olive oil, and the parsley. Lower heat to medium and cook, covered, at a medium boil, stirring occasionally, for about 1½ hours until the beans are tender. Meanwhile, in a large skillet heat the remaining ⅓ cup olive oil over low-medium heat. Add the remaining 6 cloves chopped garlic, the leeks, dandelions, and tomatoes with their juices. Cover the skillet and cook for about 45 minutes, stirring occasionally, until the dandelions are tender and the sauce is thick. Sprinkle with the crushed red pepper, oregano, and salt and pepper to taste. Stir well to mix. Taste for seasonings. Lower heat and cover to keep warm while the beans continue to cook until tender.

Cook the ziti according to package directions. Drain and add the pasta to the cooked dandelion greens. Cover and keep warm until the beans are tender. When the beans are done, mash lightly with a potato masher. Turn the cooked dandelion mixture into the pot of beans, using a rubber spatula to scrape the skillet clean. Stir well to combine. Cook for 10 minutes, stirring occasionally. Taste for seasonings.

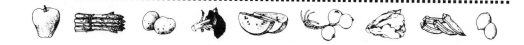

Broccoli Rabe Lasagna

SERVES 12

My love for broccoli rabe stems back to my early childhood. Most of the women in my family prepared this vitamin A-packed, traditional Italian bitter green as a side dish, as a topping for linguine, or on a sandwich with melted mozzarella cheese. It never occurred to me that this family favorite of ours would make a luscious filling for lasagna, at least not until my brother Paul told me that he saw broccoli rabe lasagna on a menu while he was vacationing. What a delicious way to combine two favorites. Try the LightLife brand Italian meatless sausage links, found in health food stores.

    1 pound lasagna noodles, cooked according to package directions
    3 large bunches broccoli rabe (about 2½ pounds)
    ¼ cup extra-virgin olive oil
    6 large cloves garlic, minced
    1 teaspoon crushed red pepper
    1 teaspoon fennel seeds
    4 links meatless sausage, crumbled with your hands
    ¼ cup water
      Salt and pepper

"Cream" Sauce:

    2 tablespoons soybean margarine (found in health food stores) or canola oil
    2 large shallots, finely chopped
      Salt and pepper
    2 tablespoons unbleached white flour
    4 cups soy milk
    ¼ cup grated Parmesan cheese or dairy-free grated "Parmesan"

Put the cooked lasagna noodles in a bowl and cover with cold water to prevent the noodles from sticking together. Trim off and discard bottom 5 inches of the broccoli rabe stems and chop the remainder into 3-inch pieces. Heat the olive oil in a large deep pot over low-medium heat. Add the garlic, crushed red pepper, fennel seeds, and meatless sausage. Cover and cook for 5 minutes, stirring occa-

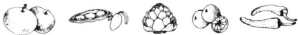

sionally, until the garlic is softened and just golden brown. Add the broccoli rabe and the water. Add salt (use a little more than usual: the bitter broccoli needs it) and a little pepper. Cover and cook for about 40 minutes, stirring occasionally, until the broccoli rabe is tender. Use tongs to turn and mix the broccoli rabe until it has cooked down enough to stir with a wooden spoon. Taste for seasonings.

Meanwhile, prepare the cream sauce: Melt the margarine or heat the canola oil in a medium pot over low heat. Add the shallots. Sprinkle with salt and pepper to taste. Cover and cook for 5 minutes, stirring occasionally, until the shallots are softened. Add the flour. Stir well to blend. Cook, uncovered, for 5 minutes, stirring frequently so that it doesn't burn. Gradually add the soy milk, stirring continuously while you pour. Cook, uncovered, over low heat for 35 minutes, stirring frequently, until the sauce is thickened slightly. Stir in the grated Parmesan cheese. Taste for seasonings.

Preheat the oven to 350 degrees. To assemble the lasagna, spray a lasagna pan with nonstick cooking spray. Drain the lasagna noodles. Arrange a single layer of 5 noodles, overlapping slightly, on the bottom of the lasagna pan. Using tongs, arrange a third of the broccoli rabe mixture evenly over the noodles. Repeat for two more layers, ending with a fourth layer of noodles. Pour the sauce evenly over the lasagna. Bake for 30 minutes to heat through. Allow to set for 5 minutes before cutting into 12 serving pieces.

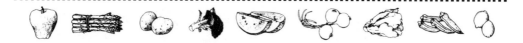

Pumpkin Squash Lasagna

SERVES 12

*My friend Rose, who is also one of the superb managers at **Claire's**, inspired me to create this wonderful autumn lasagna.*

- 1 pound lasagna noodles
- 3 tablespoons extra-virgin olive oil
- 5 large cloves garlic, minced
- 6 pounds (about) Caribbean pumpkin squash (calabaza, not American pumpkin), peeled, cut into ½-inch cubes
- ½ cup finely chopped fresh Italian flat-leaf parsley
- 10 large basil leaves, coarsely chopped
  Salt and pepper
- 3 tablespoons soybean margarine (found in health food stores)
- 1 medium sweet onion, finely chopped
- 1 large shallot, minced
- 3 tablespoons flour
- 4 cups soy milk (found in health food stores and supermarkets)
- ⅛ teaspoon nutmeg

Cook lasagna noodles according to package directions. Drain. Turn into a bowl of cold water to prevent sticking. Heat the olive oil in a large deep sauté pan over medium heat. Add the garlic, squash, parsley, basil, and salt and pepper to taste. Cover and cook for about 35 minutes, stirring occasionally, until the squash is just tender. Taste for seasonings. Remove from heat. Meanwhile, melt the margarine in a large skillet over medium heat. Add the onion and the shallot. Cover and cook for 10 minutes, stirring occasionally, until the onion has softened. Whisk in the flour, mixing to combine. Cook, stirring frequently, for 5 minutes, scraping the pan as you stir. Gradually pour in the soy milk, stirring continuously as you pour. Continue stirring until the mixture is combined. Cook, stirring occasionally, for about 25 minutes until the sauce thickens slightly. Stir in the nutmeg, and salt and pepper to taste. Remove from heat.

Preheat the oven to 350 degrees. Spray a large glass baking dish with nonstick cooking spray. Spread ½ cup of the sauce in the bottom of the prepared dish.

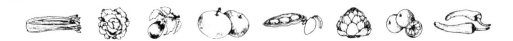

Drain the lasagna noodles. Arrange a layer of the lasagna noodles (about 5) over the sauce, overlapping slightly. Spoon one third of the squash evenly over the noodles. Spoon ½ cup of sauce over the squash. Arrange another layer of noodles over the sauce. Repeat with another two layers ending with a fourth layer of noodles, then pour the remaining sauce evenly over the noodles. Cover the baking dish with foil. Bake for 40 minutes. Allow to set for 5 minutes before serving.

Hearty Bell Pepper-"Bacon" Sauce over Gnocchi

SERVES 6 TO 8

My grandmother often made a traditional southern Italian sauce very much like this one. She served it with plump potato dumplings called gnocchi that she added during the last couple of minutes of cooking, which gave the sauce a rich creamy flavor. This makes a wonderfully satisfying sauce for any pasta. Grate a little Parmesan cheese, grind a little black pepper, and enjoy this wonderful dish.

- 4 tablespoons extra-virgin olive oil
- 1 large shallot, minced
- 1 medium leek, white part and 6 inches of pale green, finely chopped
- 6 medium cloves garlic, coarsely chopped
- 1 medium onion, finely chopped
- 3 large bell peppers (red, yellow, and/or green), seeded and coarsely chopped
- ¼ cup finely chopped fresh Italian flat-leaf parsley
- 1 6-ounce package meatless bacon, coarsely chopped (found in many supermarkets and health food stores)
  Salt and pepper
- 1 28-ounce can Italian whole peeled tomatoes, with juice, squeezed with your hands to crush
- 2 tablespoons tomato paste
- 2 cups water
- 10 large fresh basil leaves
- ⅓ cup red (sweet) vermouth
- ¼ cup pitted and chopped oil-cured black olives
- 2 pounds frozen potato gnocchi

Heat the olive oil in a large deep skillet over medium heat. Add the shallot, leek, garlic, onion, peppers, parsley, and meatless bacon. Stir in salt and pepper to taste. Cover and cook for 20 minutes, stirring occasionally, until the peppers and onions have softened and have released some of their liquids. Add the tomatoes, tomato paste, and water. Stir to mix well. Cover and bring to a boil over medium heat (this should take about 10 minutes), stirring occasionally. Lower the heat to medium-low. Cook, covered, at a medium boil, stirring occasionally, for 45 minutes. Stir in the basil, vermouth, and olives. Cover and continue cooking for 15 minutes, stirring occasionally.

Meanwhile, cook the gnocchi according to package directions. Add the cooked and drained gnocchi to the sauce. Cook, uncovered, stirring frequently, for 5 minutes until the sauce has thickened slightly. Taste for seasonings.

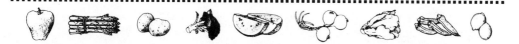

Tortellini with Green Peas, Red Onion, and Meatless Bacon

SERVES 4 TO 6

It's hard to believe that a dish this rich and luscious is also cholesterol-free. You can find tofu tortellini and meatless bacon (LightLife Foods makes the Fakin' Bacon brand) in the freezer section of health food stores.

 4 tablespoons soybean margarine (found in health food stores) or canola oil
 1 medium red (Bermuda) onion, finely chopped
 1 medium sweet onion, finely chopped
 1 6-ounce package meatless bacon, cut into ¾-inch pieces
   Salt and pepper
 3 tablespoons unbleached flour
 4 cups soy milk
12 large fresh basil leaves
 1 10-ounce package frozen petite green peas
 1 pound frozen cheese or tofu tortellini

Melt the soy margarine or heat the canola oil in a medium pot over low heat. Add the red and sweet onions. Cook and raise the heat to low-medium. Cook for 10 minutes, stirring occasionally, until the onions are softened. Add the meatless bacon. Sprinkle with salt and pepper to taste. Cover and continue cooking for 20 minutes, stirring occasionally. Sprinkle the flour over the mixture. Stir well to mix. Cover and continue cooking for 5 minutes, stirring frequently. Gradually stir in the soy milk, ½ cup at a time, stopping in between additions to mix well.

Continue cooking, uncovered, for about 10 minutes, stirring frequently, until heated through. Stir in the basil leaves and the green peas. Continue cooking for 30 minutes, stirring frequently, until the peas are heated through and the sauce has thickened slightly. Taste for seasonings. Turn off the heat, cover the pot, and keep the sauce warm while you cook the tortellini according to package directions. Drain well. Turn the tortellini into the sauce. Raise the heat to medium. Stir well to combine. Cook, stirring constantly, for 1 minute until heated through. Serve immediately.

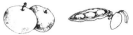

Spicy Fresh Tomato and "Cream"-Sauced Penne

SERVES 4

Tomato sauces have always been a favorite in my restaurant and in my family. This sauce gets its nice spicy flavor from hot cherry peppers and a delicious creamy texture from soy milk, and the results are truly delicious. This recipe calls for penne pasta, but the sauce is great over any pasta, tortellini, or ravioli.

3 tablespoons extra-virgin olive oil
4 large cloves garlic, finely chopped
1 large shallot, minced
1 medium leek, white part and 6 inches of pale green, finely chopped
2 hot cherry peppers, finely chopped (wash your hands immediately after handling hot peppers)
25 string beans, trimmed and cut into 1-inch pieces
5 large ripe tomatoes (red and/or yellow), cut into 1-inch cubes
½ cup finely chopped fresh Italian flat-leaf parsley
2 teaspoons dried oregano
1 teaspoon crushed red pepper
¼ teaspoon ground red pepper (cayenne)
  Salt
1 pound penne pasta
1 cup soy milk (found in most supermarkets and health food stores)

Heat the olive oil in a large deep skillet over medium heat. Add the garlic, shallot, leek, cherry peppers, and string beans. Cover and cook for 10 minutes, stirring occasionally, until the leeks are softened. Add the tomatoes, parsley, oregano, crushed red pepper, and cayenne. Sprinkle with salt. Stir well to mix. Cover and cook for 20 minutes, stirring occasionally, until the green beans are barely tender (the sauce should cook at a medium boil as the tomatoes soften).

Meanwhile, cook the pasta according to package directions while you finish the sauce: Gradually stir in the soy milk, stirring continuously as you pour. Cover and continue cooking for 10 minutes, stirring occasionally. Add salt and pepper to taste. Turn the cooked and drained pasta into a bowl. Ladle half of the sauce over the pasta. Toss to coat the pasta. Ladle the remaining sauce over the pasta. Serve immediately.

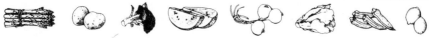

Meatless Bolognese Sauce for Rigatoni

SERVES 6 TO 8

When my father-in-law was first informed that he had to eliminate meat from his diet for medical reasons, he was overwhelmed. The idea of never enjoying his favorite foods again sent him into a depression. I was determined to return the smile to this fine man's face by preparing delicious sauces like this one. You will need to buy 2 cups of TVP (textured vegetable protein) at a health food store, and if this is a new ingredient for you, please trust me on this one. You won't regret it once you've tasted this richly flavored, protein-packed, cholesterol-free sauce.

      4 cups water
     ½ teaspoon salt
      2 cups TVP (found in health food stores)
     ¼ cup extra-virgin olive oil
      8 large cloves garlic, finely chopped
      2 medium onions, coarsely chopped
      1 35-ounce can Italian peeled tomatoes, with juice, squeezed with your
         hands to crush
      1 6-ounce can tomato paste
      3 cups water
     ½ cup dry vermouth
     ½ cup coarsely chopped fresh Italian flat-leaf parsley
      1 14-ounce can artichoke hearts, drained and sliced
     ½ cup chopped fresh basil
     ¼ teaspoon crushed red pepper
         Salt and pepper
    1½ pounds rigatoni or your favorite pasta

   In a medium covered pot, bring 4 cups of water to a boil. Add ½ teaspoon salt and the TVP. Stir well to mix. Remove from heat, and let stand, covered, for 5 minutes to absorb the water and reconstitute (puff up). Heat the olive oil in a large skillet over medium heat. Add the garlic and the onions. Cover and cook

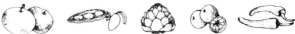

for 5 minutes, stirring occasionally, until softened but not browned. Add the tomatoes, tomato paste, water, vermouth, and parsley. Cover and bring to a boil. Remove cover and cook, uncovered, at a medium boil for 45 minutes, stirring frequently. Stir in the TVP, artichoke hearts, basil, and crushed red pepper, mixing well to combine. Stir in salt and pepper to taste. Continue cooking for 30 minutes, stirring occasionally. Taste for seasonings.

Meanwhile, cook the pasta according to package directions. Drain the pasta and turn it into a serving bowl. Ladle half of the sauce over the pasta. Toss well using two spoons. Ladle the remaining sauce over the pasta. Any extra sauce can be frozen for up to one month.

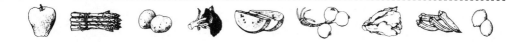

Marinara Sauce

MAKES 9 CUPS

This beautifully flavored marinara sauce makes enough for two pounds of your favorite pasta, so why not enjoy it twice by freezing half for a second delicious supper?

½ cup plus 2 tablespoons extra-virgin olive oil
2 medium sweet onions, coarsely chopped
6 large cloves garlic, coarsely chopped
½ teaspoon crushed red pepper
  Salt and pepper
2 28-ounce cans Italian peeled tomatoes, with juice, squeezed with your hands to crush
¼ cup chopped fresh Italian flat-leaf parsley
1 6-ounce can tomato paste
1 large ripe tomato, chopped, juices included
3 cups water
1 bay leaf
½ teaspoon ground red pepper (cayenne)
¼ cup fresh basil leaves

Heat the olive oil in a large pot over low-medium heat. Add the onions and garlic. Cook for 3 to 4 minutes, stirring frequently, until the onions are softened. Stir in the crushed red pepper and cook for another minute. Sprinkle with salt and pepper to taste. Stir well to mix. Add the canned tomatoes, parsley, tomato paste, ripe tomato, water, bay leaf, and cayenne. Sprinkle with salt and pepper to taste. Cover and bring to a boil over low-medium heat, stirring frequently. When it reaches a boil, remove the cover. Continue cooking, uncovered, at a low-medium boil for about 1 hour, stirring frequently, until the sauce reduces by one fourth and thickens slightly.

Coarsely chop the fresh basil. Stir the basil into the sauce, and salt and pepper to taste. Remove the bay leaf. Taste for seasonings. Serve immediately, or when the sauce cools to room temperature, freeze. Use within two months.

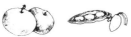

5
Entrees

- Vegetable Burgers in an Orange-Mustard Sauce
- Vegetable Burgers Calvados
- Chicken-Fried Vegetable Burgers with Sawmill Gravy
- Vegetable Burgers au Poivre
- Vegetable Burgers Sauerbraten-Style
- Ratatouille with Goat Cheese Dumplings
- Vegetable Cobbler with Parmesan-Herb Dumplings
- Vegetable Gumbo
- Curried Vegetables with Chick-peas
- Thai Vegetables with Jasmine Rice
- New England Boiled Dinner
- Vegetables Paprikas
- Vegetable Burgers in a Creamy Tarragon Sauce
- Caribbean-Style Vegetables with Brown Rice and Black Beans
- Roasted Vegetables with a Sun-Dried Tomato Aioli
- Broccoli and Garlic in Orange Sauce over Gingered Rice
- Portobello Mushrooms with Gorgonzola Cheese over Mushroom Polenta
- Portobello Mushrooms Pizzaola
- Greek Lima Beans, Artichoke Hearts, and Scallions with Orzo, Feta Cheese, and Spinach
- Zucchini Balls with Mint and Olives, Baked in Marinara Sauce
- Cajun-Style Pan-Blackened Tofu with Pepper Relish
- Tofu and Broccoli Divan
- Zucchini in Curry Sauce with Rice and Golden Raisins

- Tofu with Mushrooms Marsala
- Maryland-Style Tofu Cakes
- Tofu Cutlets Veracruz-Style
- Seitan Osso Buco-Style
- Peppers, Potatoes, and Tofu Hot Dogs
- Tofu Hot Dogs Italian-Style, with Red Peppers, Onions, and Tomatoes
- Acorn Squash Stuffed with Cornbread, Rice, Pears, Cranberries, and Pecans
- Sicilian Stuffed Eggplant Halves
- Stuffed Escarole
- Tempeh and Vegetables in Barbecue Sauce
- "Sausage"- and Broccoli-Stuffed Mushroom Caps
- Acorn Squash with Rice and Vegetable Stuffing
- Jumbo Mushroom Caps Filled with Spinach, Tofu, and Sun-Dried Tomatoes
- Artichoke Pie
- Stuffed Pepper Halves
- Spinach, Tomato, and Goat Cheese Pizzas
- Mushroom Quesadillas
- Mexican Vegetables and Pinto Beans over Yellow Rice
- Sweet and White Potato Burritos with Avocado-Jalapeño Sauce
- Black Bean Quesadillas
- Spinach Pie
- Shepherd's Pie
- Sicilian Rice Balls
- Broccoli Rabe with White Beans and Potatoes
- Nitin Pakoras
- Spinach Empanadas Gallega
- Asparagus Mini Omelettes
- Potato, "Sausage," and Mushroom Pancakes
- Corn-Crusted Parsnip, Sweet and White Potato Cakes
- Garden Paella
- Asparagus and Tofu Pancakes
- Kasha with Cabbage and Portobello Mushrooms
- Sweet Potatoes and Kidney Beans over "Sausage" and Polenta
- Stewed White Beans with Spinach, Onions, and Garlic Toasts
- Cauliflower with Angel Hair Pasta in a Light Broth with Parmesan Cheese
- Potatoes and Eggs
- Grandma McHugh's Baked Beans with Meatless Hot Dogs

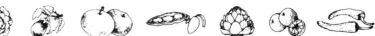

Vegetable Burgers in an Orange-Mustard Sauce

SERVES 4

A sauté is quick to prepare, yet always seems so elegant. Enjoy this special dish with Scalloped Potatoes (page 106) and Sautéed Zucchini Spears (page 112), which can both be prepared in advance and reheated for extra convenience.

3 tablespoons soybean margarine (found in health food stores) or canola oil
1 large shallot, minced
4 vegetable burgers, frozen (I like Green Giant's Harvest Burgers best for this recipe)
2 cups orange juice
⅛ teaspoon ground red pepper (cayenne)
¼ cup Dijon mustard
1 tablespoon honey
2 tablespoons arrowroot powder or cornstarch
   Salt and pepper
4 cups cooked jasmine or short-grain brown rice

Melt the margarine or heat the oil in a large deep skillet over medium heat. Add the shallot. Cover and cook for 5 minutes, stirring occasionally, until the shallots are softened. Arrange the vegetable burgers in a single layer over the shallots. Cover and cook for 3 to 4 minutes, until lightly browned, then carefully turn over and cook the other side for 3 to 4 minutes.

In a bowl, whisk together the orange juice, red pepper, mustard, and honey until well blended. Whisk in the arrowroot, and salt and pepper to taste, whisking well to combine. Pour this over the burgers. Cook for 4 to 5 minutes, occasionally moving the pan in a circular motion until the sauce thickens. Taste for seasonings. Spoon the cooked rice onto a serving platter. Spoon the vegetable burgers and the sauce over the rice. Serve immediately.

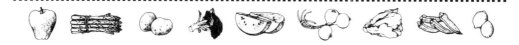

Vegetable Burgers Calvados

SERVES 4

Many years ago, Shannon Murphy, one of many marvelous cooks I have known, made a delicious dish of chicken breasts sautéed in Calvados or apple brandy. This dish substitutes vegetables for the chicken and is wonderful served with Garlic Mashed Potatoes (page 105), corn on the cob, and a green salad. I use Harvest Burgers (Green Giant) in this recipe and they can be found in the freezer section of most supermarkets or at health food stores.

    2 tablespoons extra-virgin olive oil
    1 teaspoon soybean margarine or canola oil
    2 large shallots, finely chopped
    2 large cloves garlic, finely chopped
    2 medium unpeeled apples (preferably Rome or Macintosh), cut in half,
        cored, cut into ¼-inch wedges
    4 vegetable burgers, partially defrosted
    ¼ cup Calvados (French apple brandy) or applejack
    ¾ cup soy milk
    ¾ cup rice milk (found in health food stores)
    1 tablespoon arrowroot powder or cornstarch
      Salt and pepper

Heat the oil and the butter in a large skillet over medium heat. Add the shallots, garlic, and apples. Cover and cook for 15 minutes, stirring occasionally and turning the apples so that they cook evenly. Arrange the vegetable burgers in a single layer over the apples. Pour the Calvados evenly over the burgers. Cover and cook for 3 minutes. Carefully turn the burgers, using two plastic spatulas. Pour the soy milk over the burgers. Cover and continue cooking for about 5 minutes, occasionally moving the skillet back and forth carefully and in a circular motion to mix the liquids together.

Meanwhile, in a small bowl, whisk together the rice milk, arrowroot powder, and a little salt and pepper. Pour over the burgers. Cook for 5 minutes, occasionally moving the skillet in a circular motion to mix the flavors as the sauce thickens. With a spoon, carefully stir the gravy, trying not to break the burgers, and spooning the gravy over the burgers as you mix. Taste for seasonings.

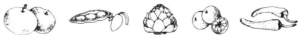

Chicken-Fried Vegetable Burgers with Sawmill Gravy

SERVES 4

Serve this southern favorite with Biscuits (page 126) and Southern-Style Green Beans (page 80).

  4 meatless burgers, defrosted (found in most supermarkets and health food stores)
  ¼ cup flour
  1 teaspoon dried thyme
     Salt and pepper
  3 tablespoons peanut oil
  2½ cups Sawmill Gravy (page 125)

Set the burgers aside to defrost until they are soft enough to dredge in flour. In a shallow bowl, combine the flour, thyme, and salt and pepper to taste. Whisk to mix. Dredge the vegetable burgers in the flour mixture, gently pressing to coat both sides evenly. Shake off excess, but make sure the burgers are heavily coated. Heat the peanut oil in a large skillet over medium-high heat. Arrange the burgers in a single layer in the hot oil. Cook the burgers for 5 minutes, without turning, then turn each burger, using two spatulas. Cook the other side for about 5 minutes until browned. Serve with Sawmill Gravy.

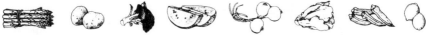

Vegetable Burgers au Poivre

SERVES 6

The frozen foods section of supermarkets across the country are now carrying a wide selection of meatless burgers. Some are made with textured soy protein and wheat gluten, which are my favorites because of their rich and "meaty" texture, and other vegetable burgers are made with nuts, vegetables, and grains. You can grill them for the quintessential American sandwich (if you choose fat-free burgers, spray both sides of the burgers with nonstick cooking spray beforehand or you will be scraping them off the grill!); you can use them for Shepherd's Pie (page 244), and for this luscious and elegant cholesterol-free adaptation of a classic French dish. I serve this lovely dish with Garlic Mashed Potatoes (page 105), Sautéed Green Beans, Carrots, and Shiitake Mushrooms (page 85), and Fresh Tomato Salad (page 54).

2 tablespoons soybean margarine (found in health food stores) or canola oil
2 tablespoons extra-virgin olive oil
3 large shallots, finely chopped
2 large cloves garlic, minced
3 tablespoons bottled steak sauce
2 tablespoons water
6 vegetable burgers, partially defrosted
1 tablespoon black and green peppercorns, coarsely cracked using a mortar and pestle
¼ cup Cognac
2 cups soy milk
2 tablespoons arrowroot powder or cornstarch
Salt and pepper

Heat the margarine and the olive oil together in a large skillet over medium heat. Add the shallots and garlic. Cook for 5 minutes, stirring occasionally, until softened. Add the steak sauce and water. Stir to combine. Cover and continue cooking for 10 minutes, stirring occasionally, as it cooks at a low boil. Arrange the vegetable burgers in a single layer in the skillet. Scatter the crushed peppercorns evenly over the burgers. Using the back of a spoon, gently press the peppercorns into the burgers. Do not crush the burgers, just push the peppercorns into the tops of the burgers. Cover and cook without disturbing for 5 minutes. Carefully turn the burgers, using a plastic spatula. Drizzle the Cognac evenly over the burgers. Cover and continue cooking for another 3 to 5 minutes, until the burgers are fully heated in the center. You can check this by inserting a fork into the center of the burger: If the tines of the fork are hot when you remove the fork, then the burgers are ready for you to proceed. If not, try again in a minute or two.

In a separate bowl combine the soy milk with the arrowroot. Sprinkle with salt and pepper to taste. Whisk well to combine. Pour this mixture all at once over the burgers. Raise the heat to medium-high. Carefully shake the skillet back and forth and in a circular pattern for about 1½ to 2 minutes to move the sauce around the burgers until the sauce thickens slightly. Taste for seasonings. Serve immediately.

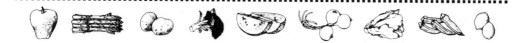

Vegetable Burgers
Sauerbraten-Style

SERVES 4

*My friend and fellow food aficionada Lucy Bouck, who lives in a German neigh-
borhood in St. Louis, makes the beef sauerbraten that served as the inspiration
for this vegetarian version. It is a traditional German dish, served over noodles.
Serve sauerbraten with German-Style Red Cabbage and Apples (page 90).*

- 4 meatless burgers, defrosted (found in most supermarkets and in health food stores)
- ¼ cup flour
- ¼ teaspoon ground cloves
  Salt and pepper
- 3 tablespoons canola oil
- 2 medium sweet onions, coarsely chopped
- ½ cup apple cider vinegar
- ¼ cup red wine
- ½ cup firmly packed brown sugar
- 1 tablespoon finely grated lemon zest
- ½ lemon, squeezed, about 2 tablespoons juice
- ¼ cup water
- 1 bay leaf
- ½ cup crumbled ginger snaps
- ½ pound wide noodles
- 2 tablespoons soybean margarine (found in health food stores), cut into tiny pieces, or canola oil
- 1 tablespoon caraway seeds

Defrost the vegetable burgers until they are soft enough to dredge in the flour.
In a shallow bowl, combine the flour, cloves, and salt and pepper to taste. Whisk
to mix. Dredge the vegetable burgers in the flour mixture, pressing down to coat
both sides of the burgers evenly. Shake off excess. Heat the oil in a large deep
skillet over medium heat. Add the onions. Cover and cook for 5 minutes, stirring

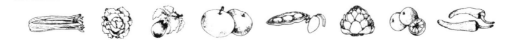

occasionally, until the onions are softened. Arrange the coated vegetable burgers over the onions. Cover and cook for 3 minutes. Turn the burgers and cook the other side for 3 minutes until lightly browned.

In a bowl, combine the cider vinegar, red wine, brown sugar, lemon zest, lemon juice, water, bay leaf, ginger snaps, and salt and pepper to taste. Whisk together until well blended. Pour this over the burgers. Cover and cook for 10 minutes, stirring occasionally, until the sauce is thick and bubbling. Taste for seasonings. Remove the bay leaf. Cook the noodles according to package directions. Drain. Return to the cooking pot. Scatter the margarine or drizzle the oil over the noodles. Toss to coat the noodles, using two spoons, until the margarine melts. Add the caraway seeds and salt and pepper to taste, tossing to mix evenly. Turn the noodles onto one side of a serving platter. Arrange the burgers and their juices alongside the noodles.

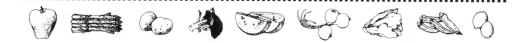

Ratatouille with Goat Cheese Dumplings

SERVES 6

Goat cheese melted over ratatouille is one of the most wonderful flavor combinations I know of. And any leftovers make a great sandwich filling on a sturdy Italian or French bread, served heated or at room temperature. Bring along a fork.

  4 tablespoons extra-virgin olive oil
  2 medium sweet onions, cut into thick ribs
  3 large cloves garlic, sliced
  2 medium eggplants, cut into ½-inch cubes
    Salt and pepper
  2 medium zucchini, cut into ¼-inch slices
  2 yellow summer squash, cut into ¼-inch slices
  2 medium potatoes, peeled, cut in half lengthwise, then into ½-inch slices
  6 medium button mushrooms, quartered
  2 medium ripe tomatoes, coarsely chopped
  1 teaspoon dried thyme
 10 large fresh basil leaves

Goat Cheese Dumplings:

  5 ounces goat cheese, softened to room temperature
  1 teaspoon dried thyme
  3 tablespoons flour
  2 tablespoons soy milk
  1 egg or egg substitute, lightly beaten
    Salt and pepper

Heat the oil in a large deep sauté pan over medium heat. Add the onions, garlic, and eggplant. Sprinkle with salt and pepper. Cover and cook for 20 minutes, stirring occasionally, until the eggplant has softened. Add the zucchini, summer squash, potatoes, mushrooms, tomatoes, thyme, and basil. Cook at a low boil, uncovered, for 30 minutes, stirring occasionally, until the potatoes are tender. Taste for seasonings.

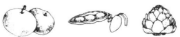

Meanwhile, prepare the goat cheese dumplings: Combine the goat cheese, thyme, flour, soy milk, egg, and salt and pepper to taste in a bowl. Mix well to blend, beating with a wooden spoon until smooth. Taste for seasonings. When the vegetables are just tender, drop the dumplings by teaspoonfuls over the simmering ratatouille. Cover and cook for 10 minutes until heated through, occasionally basting the dumplings with the ratatouille, using a spoon.

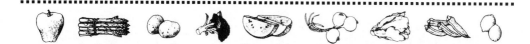

Vegetable Cobbler with Parmesan-Herb Dumplings

SERVES 6

There is something ever so comforting about coming home to the wonderful aromas that fill the kitchen when a pot of vegetable cobbler is simmering on the stove. Sometimes when I make a cobbler, I walk out the front door and come right in through the back door so that I, too, can come home to the aromas. Try it.

3 tablespoons soybean margarine (**found in health food stores**) **or canola oil**
2 medium sweet onions, coarsely chopped
3 medium carrots, peeled, cut into ½-inch slices
3 ribs celery, cut into ½-inch slices
2 medium parsnips, peeled, cut into ½-inch slices
1 medium cauliflower, cored and coarsely chopped
3 medium potatoes, peeled, cut into ½-inch cubes
  Salt and pepper
1 cup frozen tiny green peas
  Fresh corn kernels cut from 2 large ears of corn (about 2 cups)
¼ pound button mushrooms, quartered
1 teaspoon dried thyme
1 teaspoon dried sage
¼ cup coarsely chopped fresh Italian flat-leaf parsley
1 bay leaf
3 cups water
1 cup cooked baby lima beans (frozen are fine)
3 cups soy milk (found in most supermarkets and health food stores)
3 tablespoons flour

Melt the margarine or heat the oil in a 7- or 8-quart Dutch oven or deep sauté pan over low heat. Add the onions, carrots, celery, parsnips, cauliflower, and potatoes. Sprinkle with salt and pepper. Cover and cook for 25 minutes, stirring occasionally until the vegetables have softened and have released some of their liquids. Stir in the peas, corn, mushrooms, thyme, sage, parsley, bay leaf, and

    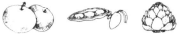

water. Cover and bring to a boil (this should take about 8 minutes). Lower the heat to medium-low and cook, covered, at a low boil for 25 minutes, stirring occasionally, until the carrots are crisp-tender. Stir in the cooked lima beans. In a bowl, whisk together the soy milk and flour, whisking until smooth. Gradually pour the milk-flour mixture into the vegetables, stirring continuously as you pour. Cook, uncovered, for 30 minutes, stirring frequently until the sauce thickens slightly. Remove the bay leaf. Meanwhile, prepare the Parmesan-Herb Dumplings:

Parmesan-Herb Dumplings:

 2 cups flour
 2 teaspoons baking powder
 ⅛ teaspoon salt
 3 tablespoons grated Parmesan cheese
 ¼ teaspoon black pepper
 1 teaspoon dried thyme
 1 teaspoon dried sage
 ¼ teaspoon ground red pepper (cayenne)
 ¼ cup Spectrum spread (found in health food stores), or vegetable shortening
 1 egg or egg substitute, lightly beaten
 ¾ cup soy milk

Measure the flour, baking powder, and salt into a bowl. Sift this into another bowl. Whisk in the Parmesan, black pepper, thyme, sage, and red pepper. Cut in the Spectrum spread using two butter knives until the mixture resembles coarse cornmeal. In a separate bowl, combine the egg and the soy milk. Whisk together to blend. Pour this over the flour mixture, all at once. Stir to combine into a sticky dough.

When the cobbler vegetables are tender, drop the dumplings by teaspoonsful on *top* of the simmering cobbler. Cover and cook for 15 minutes, occasionally basting the dumplings with the cooking liquid from the cobbler, using a baster or a spoon. After the 15 minutes the dumplings should be set enough to stir the cobbler, so the dumplings can finish cooking *in* the cobbler. Cover and continue cooking for another 15 minutes until the dumplings are cooked. Test by cutting one dumpling in half to check for doneness. It should be firm inside with no uncooked batter.

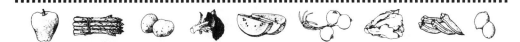

Vegetable Gumbo

SERVES 8

My husband and I have always loved the rich and spicy flavors of a hearty gumbo, the Creole stew that bursts with the flavors of herbed tomatoes, sausage, okra, and hot sauce. Serve this luscious, cholesterol-free gumbo with Candied Sweet Potatoes (page 108) and cornbread for a very satisfying down-home meal.

     3 tablespoons olive oil
     2 medium onions, chopped
     2 large cloves garlic, chopped
     3 large green bell peppers, seeded and chopped
    10 green beans, cut into 1-inch pieces
     4 large ribs celery with leaves, chopped
    ½ pound (about 30 pods) okra, sliced into ½-inch pieces
     3 ounces meatless bacon (found in health food stores)
    ½ cup chopped fresh Italian flat-leaf parsley
     5 scallions, white part and 3 inches of green, cut into ½-inch pieces
     3 large tomatoes, chopped
        Salt and pepper
     1 35-ounce can Italian whole peeled tomatoes, with juice, squeezed with
        your hands to crush
     1 teaspoon Old Bay seasoning
     1 teaspoon paprika (hot is best)
    ¼ teaspoon ground red pepper (cayenne)
    ½ teaspoon dried thyme
    ½ teaspoon fennel seeds
    ½ teaspoon dried rosemary
     1 12-ounce package meatless Italian sausage (found in health food stores),
        cut into 1-inch pieces
     1 cup cold water
     2 tablespoons cornstarch
     2 to 3 dashes Tabasco
     8 cups cooked brown rice

    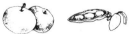

Heat the oil in a large pot over medium heat. Add the onions, garlic, bell peppers, green beans, celery, okra, meatless bacon, parsley, scallions, and fresh tomatoes. Sprinkle lightly with salt and pepper. Stir to combine and to coat with the oil. Cover and cook over medium heat for 10 minutes, stirring occasionally. Add the canned tomatoes in juice, Old Bay seasoning, paprika, cayenne, thyme, fennel, rosemary, and meatless sausage. Stir well to mix. Cover and cook over medium heat. After it begins to boil, cook for about 30 minutes, stirring occasionally, until the vegetables are tender. In a separate bowl, whisk together the cold water and the cornstarch until smooth. Pour this into the gumbo, stirring to mix well. Raise the heat to medium-high and bring to a boil. Lower the heat to medium and cook, uncovered, at a low boil for 15 minutes, stirring frequently until the soup has thickened. Stir in the Tabasco. Taste for seasonings. Spread the cooked rice in a large serving platter. Spoon the gumbo over the rice. Serve immediately.

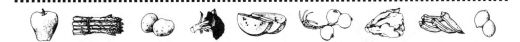

Curried Vegetables with Chick-peas

SERVES 6

Serve this aromatic, substantial vegetable stew with Basmati Rice with Green Peas and Pine Nuts (page 119). Classic Indian vegetable curries are a natural for any vegetarian diet.

      2 tablespoons peanut oil
      3 medium sweet onions, cut into ½ inch rings
      3 tablespoons curry powder
      ½ teaspoon ground cinnamon
      3 medium carrots, peeled and cut on the diagonal into ½-inch slices
      ½ medium cauliflower, cored and coarsely chopped
         Salt and pepper
      1 bay leaf
      2 medium bell peppers (1 red and 1 green), seeded and coarsely chopped
      ¼ pound (about 15 large) green beans, cut into ½-inch pieces
      2 medium sweet potatoes, peeled and cut into 1-inch cubes
      1 medium white potato, peeled and cut into 1-inch cubes
      3 medium zucchini, cut into ½-inch slices
      2 large ripe tomatoes, coarsely chopped
      3 cups water
         Fresh corn kernels cut from 2 large ears of corn (about 2 cups), *or* frozen kernels
      1 large Granny Smith apple, coarsely chopped
      2 cups cooked chick-peas
      2 tablespoons cornstarch
      ½ cup water
      1 cup frozen green peas
      ¼ teaspoon ground red pepper (cayenne)

Heat the oil in a large pot over medium heat. Add the onions. Stir to coat with the oil. Sprinkle with the curry powder and cinnamon. Stir well to mix. Add the

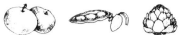

carrots and cauliflower. Sprinkle with salt and pepper. Add the bay leaf. Cover and cook for 10 minutes, stirring occasionally. Add the peppers and green beans. Cover and continue cooking for 5 minutes, stirring frequently. Add the sweet and white potatoes, zucchini, and tomatoes. Add the water and stir well to combine. Cover, raise the heat to medium-high. Bring to a boil, then lower the heat to medium. Cook at a low-medium boil for about 25 minutes, stirring occasionally, until the potatoes are nearly tender.

Stir in the corn, apple, and the chick-peas. Raise the heat to medium-high, and cook, uncovered, for 2 minutes, stirring occasionally. In a separate bowl, whisk together the cornstarch with the water until smooth. Pour this into the pot, stirring well to combine. Continue cooking at a medium boil for 2 minutes, stirring occasionally, until the mixture thickens slightly. Stir in the green peas and the ground red pepper. Continue cooking for 1 minute, stirring frequently. Taste for seasonings. Remove the bay leaf.

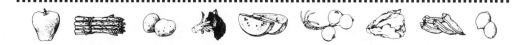

Thai Vegetables with Jasmine Rice

SERVES 6

When it comes to varieties of cuisine, New York is the place to be. That's where we first experienced Thai food. We immediately fell in love with the interesting combination of hot, spicy, and sweet flavors. This dish is delicious, but it is fairly hot. If you want a milder version, use ½ to 1 Thai chili pepper. Most supermarkets now carry a substantial variety of chili peppers, both fresh and dry. Thai chilies are thin, short (about 1 inch) red peppers, and very potent.

- 2 tablespoons peanut oil
- 2 large cloves garlic, minced
- ½-inch piece fresh ginger, peeled and finely grated
- 1 large sweet onion, coarsely chopped
- 2 Thai chili peppers or jalapeños, finely chopped (wash your hands immediately after handling the hot peppers)
- 16 green beans, trimmed and cut into ½-inch pieces
- 1 large green bell pepper, seeded and coarsely chopped
- 2 medium sweet potatoes, peeled and cut into 1-inch pieces
- 2 medium white potatoes, peeled and cut into 1-inch pieces
- 4 large ripe tomatoes, chopped (include the juices)
- Salt and pepper
- 3 limes, squeezed, about 6 tablespoons juice
- 1 14-ounce can unsweetened coconut milk
- 2 medium zucchini, cut into ½-inch slices
- 1 medium yellow summer squash, cut into ½-inch slices
- 4 scallions, white part and 3 inches of green, cut into thin slices
- Fresh corn kernels cut from 2 large ears of corn (about 1½ cups), *or* frozen kernels
- ½ cup coarsely chopped fresh basil leaves
- 1¼ cups finely chopped broccoli florets
- 6 cups cooked jasmine or basmati rice (found in the rice section of most supermarkets)

Heat the oil in a large pot over medium heat. Add the garlic, ginger, onion, and chili peppers. Cook, stirring frequently, for 3 minutes. Add the green beans, bell pepper, sweet and white potatoes, and tomatoes. Sprinkle with salt and pepper. Cover and cook for 10 minutes, stirring occasionally. Add the lime juice and the coconut milk. Stir well to combine. Raise the heat to medium high. Cover and bring to a low boil, then reduce the heat to medium. Push the potatoes down into the liquid. Cover and continue cooking at a low-medium boil for 10 to 12 minutes, stirring occasionally, until the string beans and the potatoes are crisp-tender. Add the zucchini, yellow squash, scallions, and corn. Cover and continue cooking for about 15 minutes, stirring occasionally, until the zucchini is tender. Stir in the basil and broccoli florets. Cover and continue cooking for 3 minutes, stirring occasionally, until the broccoli is tender. Taste for seasonings. Serve hot over the cooked rice.

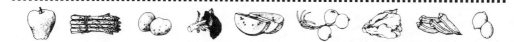

New England Boiled Dinner

SERVES 8

The veggie hot dogs and veggie back bacon give this lovely, one-pot meal a familiar, smoked flavor—and they are fat free. Enjoy this hearty stew with rye bread and good, grainy mustard for a satisfying and healthy dinner.

- 5 teaspoons extra-virgin olive oil
- 1 small head savoy cabbage, chopped
  Salt and pepper
- 3 medium carrots, cut into 1½-inch chunks
- 3 medium parsnips, cut into 1½-inch chunks
- 3 ribs celery, cut into 1½-inch chunks
- 1 cup coarsely chopped fresh Italian flat-leaf parsley
- 3 quarts water
- ½ teaspoon dried sage
- ½ teaspoon dried thyme
- 1 teaspoon fennel seeds
- 1 small butternut squash, peeled and cut into 1½-inch pieces
- 3 medium red-skinned potatoes, quartered
- 3 ears fresh corn on the cob, each cut into four pieces
- 6 fat-free veggie dogs
- 3 oz. (½ package) veggie back bacon (Yves brand, found in health food stores)
- 2 pounds sauerkraut

Heat the oil in an 8-quart sauté pan or an 8-quart soup pot over low-medium heat. Add the cabbage and sprinkle with salt and pepper. Cover and cook for 15 minutes, stirring occasionally. Add carrots, parsnips, celery, parsley, and water. Stir well to mix. Raise the heat to high, cover, and bring to a boil, then reduce the heat to medium. Add the sage, thyme, and fennel. Stir to mix well. Cook, covered, at a medium boil for 30 minutes, stirring occasionally. Add the butternut squash and potatoes. Continue cooking, covered, for 10 minutes, stirring occasionally. Add the corn and continue to cook, stirring occasionally, for 10 minutes until the potatoes and squash are tender. Add the veggie dogs, veggie bacon, and sauerkraut. Stir well to mix. Continue cooking, covered, for 2 to 3 minutes until the sauerkraut is heated through.

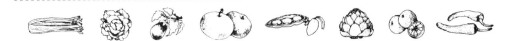

Vegetables Paprikas

SERVES 6

My sister-in-law's grandmother Betty Stevens is of Hungarian descent. This is just one of the many recipes Betty has kindly shared with me over the years. She made me promise that I would stress to you the importance of using good Hungarian paprika, so please do. I wouldn't like to disappoint Betty!

  3 tablespoons olive oil
  3 medium onions, cut in half, then into thick ribs
  1 large red (Bermuda) onion, coarsely chopped
  4 medium carrots, peeled and cut on the diagonal into ¼-inch slices
  1 large head savoy cabbage or green cabbage (about 2 pounds), cored, cut into quarters, then coarsely chopped
10 medium button mushrooms, cut into thick slices
  3 tablespoons Hungarian paprika
    Salt and pepper
 ⅓ cup red wine
  1 cup low-fat sour cream
  1 pound wide noodles, cooked according to package directions

Heat the olive oil in an large pot over medium heat. Add the onions, cover, and cook for 10 minutes, stirring occasionally. Add the carrots, cabbage, and mushrooms. Turn to coat, using tongs. Cook for 15 minutes, turning occasionally, using tongs. Stir in the paprika, salt and pepper to taste, and the red wine. Stir to coat evenly. Cover and cook for 25 minutes, stirring occasionally, until the cabbage is tender. Stir in the sour cream, mixing well to combine. Cook for 3 minutes, stirring occasionally. Taste for seasonings. Serve over the noodles.

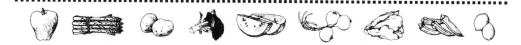

Vegetable Burgers in a Creamy Tarragon Sauce

SERVES 4

I use Green Giant's Harvest Burgers for this recipe because of their meaty texture and mild flavor, which goes nicely with the French-inspired sauce. Serve with Sweet Cinnamon Carrots (page 93), Garlic Mashed Potatoes (page 105), and Brussels Sprouts in Lemon Vinaigrette (page 88).

- 3 tablespoons soybean margarine (found in health food stores) or canola oil
- 2 large shallots, minced
- 4 vegetable burgers, frozen
- ½ cup dry white wine
- 2 teaspoons dried tarragon or 1½ tablespoons chopped fresh
- 2 cups soy milk
- 2 tablespoons arrowroot or cornstarch
- Salt and pepper

Melt the margarine or heat the oil in a large nonstick skillet over medium heat. Add the shallots. Cook for 3 minutes, stirring occasionally, until softened. Arrange the vegetable burgers in a single layer in the skillet. Cover and cook on each side for 4 minutes or until lightly browned. Pour the wine evenly over the burgers and sprinkle the tarragon evenly over the burgers. Cover and cook for about 5 minutes until the wine reduces by half. Turn the burgers over. Meanwhile, put the soy milk into a bowl. Whisk in the arrowroot until smooth. Whisk in salt and pepper to taste. Pour the milk mixture all at once over the burgers. Move the skillet in a circular motion for 2 to 3 minutes until the soy milk is heated through and the sauce has thickened slightly. Taste for seasonings. Serve immediately.

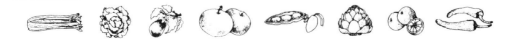

Caribbean-Style Vegetables with Brown Rice and Black Beans

SERVES 6

Shannon Murphy, one of the finest chefs I have known, always returned from her vacations with new ideas for delicious dishes that I could adapt to my vegetarian diet both at home and in my restaurant. This combination remains one of my favorites.

  3 tablespoons soybean margarine (found in health food stores) or canola oil
  1 medium red (Bermuda) onion, coarsely chopped
  3 large cloves garlic, minced
  2 to 3 pounds Caribbean pumpkin squash (calabaza; *not* American pumpkin), peeled and cut into ¼-inch cubes
  2 medium sweet potatoes, peeled and cut into ½-inch cubes
    Salt and pepper
  2 ripe plantains, peeled and cut into ½-inch slices
  ¼ cup coarsely chopped fresh cilantro
  2 limes, squeezed, about 4 tablespoons juice
 12 ounces black beans, picked over for stones
  3 quarts water
  1 bay leaf
  2 cups brown rice

Melt the margarine or heat the oil in a large, deep skillet over low-medium heat. Add the onion, garlic, squash, sweet potatoes, and salt and pepper to taste. Cover and cook for about 30 minutes, stirring occasionally, until the squash and potatoes are just tender. Stir in the plantains, cilantro, and lime juice. Cover and continue cooking for 5 minutes, stirring occasionally, until the plantains are tender.

Meanwhile, measure the beans and water into a 6-quart pot. Cover and bring to a boil over high heat. Add the bay leaf and lower the heat to medium. Cook, covered, at a medium boil for 1 hour, stirring occasionally. Stir in the brown rice, cover, and lower the heat to medium-low. Continue cooking at a low-medium boil for another 45 minutes, stirring occasionally, until the beans and rice are tender. Remove the bay leaf. Stir in salt and pepper to taste. Spoon the rice and beans into a large serving platter. Spoon the squash mixture and its juices over the rice. Serve immediately.

Roasted Vegetables with a Sun-Dried Tomato Aioli

SERVES 8

The aioli for this dish is a provençal garlic mayonnaise blended with sun-dried tomatoes. It is luscious, yet quite simple to make, and I love to make a meal by dipping a beautiful combination of vegetables into it.

  2 medium onions, quartered
  3 large cloves garlic, cut in fourths, lengthwise
  2 medium potatoes, peeled and cut into ½-inch slices
  3 medium carrots, peeled, cut in half lengthwise, then cut into ¼-inch lengthwise slices
18 string beans, trimmed
  6 large mushrooms, cut in half, lengthwise
  1 medium zucchini, cut into 1-inch slices
  6 scallions, white part and 6 inches of green, coarsely chopped
  6 baby artichokes, cut in half lengthwise
 ½ fresh lemon
 ½ pound thin asparagus, trimmed
  3 tablespoons extra-virgin olive oil
  1 tablespoon water
  2 teaspoons dried thyme
    Salt and pepper

Sun-Dried Tomato Aioli:

 ½ cup non-dairy, low-fat, or fat-free mayonnaise
  1 large clove garlic, minced
 ¼ cup chopped, drained, oil-packed sun-dried tomatoes
 ½ lemon, squeezed, about 2 tablespoons juice
    Salt and pepper

Preheat the oven to 400 degrees. Spray a large roasting pan with cooking oil spray. Place the onions, garlic, potatoes, carrots, string beans, mushrooms, zuc-

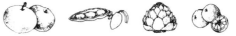

chini, and scallions in a large bowl. Rub the cut side of the artichoke halves with the lemon half. Add the artichokes and asparagus to the bowl. Toss to mix, using two spoons. Drizzle 1 tablespoon of the olive oil evenly over the vegetables. Toss well to coat. Repeat with the remaining 2 tablespoons of olive oil. Add the water. Toss well to coat. Sprinkle with thyme, and salt and pepper to taste over the vegetables. Toss well to coat. Taste for seasonings. Turn into the prepared roasting pan. Cover tightly with foil. Bake for 55 minutes, then remove the foil and continue baking, uncovered, for 10 minutes or until the vegetables are tender.

While the vegetables are roasting, prepare the sun-dried tomato aioli: Place the mayonnaise, garlic, tomatoes, and lemon juice into a blender. Cover and pulse to blend, 15 to 20 times, stopping to scrape down the sides using a rubber spatula after every 2 to 3 pulses, until the mixture is fairly smooth. Stir in salt and pepper to taste. Serve the aioli with the vegetables for dipping.

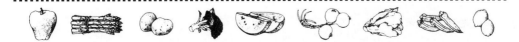

Broccoli and Garlic in Orange Sauce over Gingered Rice

SERVES 6

Broccoli, garlic, brown rice, and ginger are four delicious and healthy ingredients, and they make an excellent combination in this wonderful Asian-inspired dish. I like to set aside a little ginger rice for the next day's breakfast—it's delicious topped with brown sugar and soy milk.

Gingered Rice:

4½ cups water
  2 cups brown rice
  1 1-inch piece fresh gingerroot, peeled and finely minced
    Salt and pepper

Broccoli and Garlic in Orange Sauce:

  1 large bunch broccoli, bottom 1 inch of stems discarded
  3 tablespoons peanut oil
  6 large cloves garlic, coarsely chopped
  3 large red bell peppers, seeded and cut into ½-inch ribs
    Salt and pepper
 ¼ cup cider vinegar
 ½ cup freshly squeezed orange juice (about ½ large orange)
  2 tablespoons honey
  1 tablespoon pure vanilla extract
 ⅛ teaspoon ground red pepper (cayenne)
  1 tablespoon arrowroot powder or cornstarch

Bring the water to a boil in a medium covered pot over high heat. Stir in the brown rice and ginger. Sprinkle with salt and pepper to taste. Stir well to mix. Lower the heat to medium. Cover and cook at a low boil for 45 minutes until the rice is tender. Taste for seasonings. Meanwhile, peel the thick skin from the broccoli stems using a potato peeler. Cut off about 4 inches of stem from the broccoli, leaving about an inch or so attached to the florets. Cut the stems into ¼-inch diagonal slices. Place the cut stems into a bowl. Cut the florets with attached stems into thin spears. Place in a separate bowl.

Heat the peanut oil in a large deep sauté pan over medium heat. Add the garlic, peppers, and broccoli stems. Sprinkle with salt and pepper. Cook for 15 minutes, stirring frequently. Add the broccoli floret spears. Cook for 7 to 10 minutes, stirring frequently, until crisp-tender.

Meanwhile, in a small bowl, whisk together the cider vinegar, orange juice, honey, vanilla, and red pepper until well blended. Whisk in the cornstarch until well blended. Whisk in salt and pepper to taste. Stir all at once into the broccoli. Stir well to mix. Cook for 5 minutes, stirring frequently, until the sauce thickens. Taste for seasonings. Spoon the broccoli and sauce onto one side of a large platter, and the rice onto the other side of the platter.

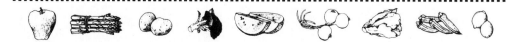

Portobello Mushrooms with Gorgonzola Cheese over Mushroom Polenta

SERVES 6

Our friends Susan and Raymond Wilson share with Frank and me a love for fresh, homemade foods, and also for big, meaty-textured portobello mushrooms. They are always on the menu whenever we share a dinner.

> 6 large portobello mushroom caps, cut into ⅓-inch slices
> 2 tablespoons extra-virgin olive oil
> 3 large cloves garlic, finely chopped
> 1 large shallot, minced
> ¼ cup finely chopped fresh Italian flat-leaf parsley
> 10 large fresh basil leaves
> Salt and pepper
> 4 ounces crumbled Gorgonzola cheese

Mushroom Polenta:

> 9 cups water
> 8 medium button mushrooms, coarsely chopped
> 2 cups white cornmeal
> ½ cup shredded mozzarella cheese
> Salt and pepper

Preheat the oven to 400 degrees. Place the portobello mushrooms in a bowl. Drizzle the olive oil over the mushrooms. Toss well to coat evenly, using two spoons. Add the garlic, shallot, parsley, and basil. Sprinkle with salt and pepper to taste. Toss well to mix. Spray a baking dish with nonstick cooking spray. Turn the mushrooms into the prepared baking dish, using a rubber spatula to scrape the bowl. Bake for about 25 minutes, stirring occasionally, until the mushrooms are just tender. Remove the mushrooms from the oven. Keep the oven on. Scatter the Gorgonzola cheese evenly over the top. Set aside.

Prepare the polenta: Bring the water to a boil in a medium covered pot over high heat. Add the button mushrooms. Cover and cook for 2 minutes, stirring occasionally. Put on a pair of oven mitts to protect your hands from the steam while cooking the polenta. Gradually pour in the cornmeal in a thin stream, continuously whisking until the mixture is smooth. Lower the heat to medium and continue whisking at a medium boil for 2 minutes. Remove from the heat. Stir in the mozzarella cheese and salt and pepper to taste. Turn the polenta into a large baking dish. Spoon the portobello mushrooms, juices, and Gorgonzola cheese over the polenta. Set the polenta in the oven and bake for 10 minutes.

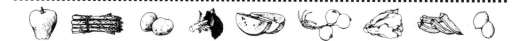

Portobello Mushrooms Pizzaola

SERVES 6

I serve this luscious ragout over linguine noodles, along with side dishes of Broccoli with Garlic Chips (page 87).

    2 tablespoons extra-virgin olive oil
    1 tablespoon extra-virgin olive oil
    3 large cloves garlic, finely chopped
    2 medium sweet onions, cut in half lengthwise, then sliced into ½-inch ribs
   12 ounces portobello mushroom caps, cut into 1 inch slices
    ¼ cup red wine
      Salt and pepper
    2 medium tomatoes, cut in half, then sliced into ½-inch wedges
    1 28-ounce can Italian whole peeled tomatoes in juice
    1 tablespoon tomato paste
    ½ cup water
    1 teaspoon dried oregano
    1 pound linguine
      Freshly grated Parmesan cheese (optional)

Heat oil and butter in a large pot over medium heat. Add the garlic and onions. Cook for 10 minutes, stirring occasionally, until the onions are softened and well coated with the oil. Add the mushroom caps and the wine. Sprinkle lightly with salt and pepper. Cook for 5 minutes, stirring occasionally, until the mushrooms begin to release their liquids. Add the fresh tomatoes and their juices, the canned tomatoes, tomato paste, water, and oregano. Raise the heat to medium-high and bring the sauce to a boil. Reduce the heat to medium, and cook at a medium boil for 30 minutes, stirring occasionally, until the mushrooms are tender and the sauce tastes rich and flavorful. Taste for seasonings.

Keep the sauce warm while you cook the pasta according to package directions. Drain the pasta and return the pasta to the pot. Spoon about half of the sauce and mushrooms over the noodles. Using two spoons, toss the sauce and the noodles to coat well. Turn into a serving bowl and spoon the remaining sauce over the top. Serve with freshly grated Parmesan cheese and additional pepper on top.

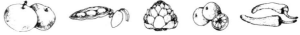

Greek Lima Beans, Artichoke Hearts, and Scallions with Orzo, Feta Cheese, and Spinach

SERVES 8

My neighbor Alice Samaras is one of the finest Greek cooks I know, and she always prepares one delicious dish after another during my visits. Alice was my inspiration for this flavorful dish, which uses traditional Greek ingredients in a very American way.

- 3 tablespoons olive oil
- 2 medium onions, minced
- 6 large cloves garlic, minced
- 6 scallions, white part and 4 inches of green, chopped
- 1 tablespoon dried dillweed or 3 tablespoons chopped fresh dill
- 1 14-ounce can artichoke hearts, drained and sliced
- 1 10-ounce bag spinach, washed and coarsely chopped
- 1 pound frozen lima beans, defrosted
- 1 pound orzo pasta, cooked according to package directions
  Salt and pepper
- ½ cup reserved cooking liquid from pasta
- 4 ounces feta cheese, crumbled

Heat the oil in a large deep skillet over medium heat. Add the onions, garlic, and scallions. Cover and cook for 15 minutes, stirring occasionally, until the onions are softened. Add the dillweed, artichoke hearts, spinach, and lima beans. Cover and cook for 15 minutes, stirring occasionally, until the spinach is tender and the lima beans are heated through. Stir in the cooked orzo, salt and pepper to taste, the reserved cooking liquid, and the feta cheese, mixing well to coat the pasta. Cover and cook for 10 minutes, stirring occasionally. Taste for seasonings.

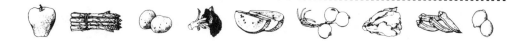

Zucchini Balls with Mint and Olives, Baked in Marinara Sauce

SERVES 6

*My aunt Louise was a model housewife and, boy, did she work hard. Her love for her work was obvious from the way she kept her home and certainly by the way she cooked. You could always depend on Aunt Louise to bring to any family gathering a batch of her wonderful Butterballs (page 281), and usually also a delicious dish flavored with fresh mint, an herb she loved. Aunt Louise was always talking about food with me and I loved her cooking. After I opened **Claire's Corner Copia**, like other beloved family members she would come in to help in the kitchen and to share recipes. This is one of them.*

4 medium zucchini, trimmed and cut into 1-inch cubes
2 tablespoons extra-virgin olive oil
2 large cloves garlic, minced
1 medium onion, minced
1 medium red bell pepper, seeded and minced
¼ cup finely chopped fresh Italian flat-leaf parsley
1 rib celery with leaves, minced
　Salt and pepper
2 teaspoons dried mint or 2 tablespoons finely minced fresh
3 cups plain dry bread crumbs
1 tablespoon finely grated lemon zest
¼ cup pitted, chopped, oil-cured black olives
3 tablespoons grated Romano cheese
2 eggs or equivalent egg substitute, lightly beaten
4 cups Marinara Sauce (page 178)

Bring a covered pot of lightly salted water to a boil over high heat. Add the zucchini. Cover and cook for about 5 minutes, until the zucchini are soft. Drain in a colander. Turn into a large bowl. Mash the zucchini with a spoon and set aside. Heat the olive oil in a skillet over low-medium heat. Add the garlic, onion, bell pepper, parsley, and celery. Sprinkle with salt and pepper to taste. Cover and

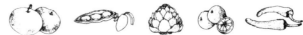

cook for 15 minutes, stirring occasionally, until the vegetables are tender and have released some of their liquids. Remove from the heat and add to the zucchini. Stir in the mint, bread crumbs, lemon zest, olives, grated cheese, and eggs. Stir to mix thoroughly. Taste for seasonings.

Preheat the oven to 400 degrees. Spoon 2 cups of the marinara sauce into a large glass baking dish. Scoop ¼ cup measures of the zucchini mixture into your hand. Roll into a ball. Place the zucchini ball in the baking dish. Repeat, using all of the zucchini mixture (about 21 balls), arranging them in a single layer over the marinara sauce. Spoon the remaining 2 cups of marinara sauce over the zucchini balls. Cover the dish tightly with foil. Bake for 1 hour or until the zucchini balls are hot and the sauce is bubbling. Serve immediately.

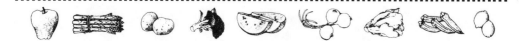

Cajun-Style Pan-Blackened Tofu with Pepper Relish

SERVES 6

If you like hot and spicy foods, then you'll love the full flavors of this New Orleans-style pan-blackened dish. The colorful pepper relish spooned on top of each tofu cutlet tempers the "fire" yet complements the rich flavors. Serve this dish with Garlic Mashed Potatoes (page 105) and Sautéed Green Beans, Carrots, and Shiitake Mushrooms (page 85).

2 pounds firm tofu, drained and cut lengthwise into ¼-inch slices
2 tablespoons flour
1 teaspoon dried thyme
1 teaspoon dried oregano
1 teaspoon ground red pepper (cayenne)
1 teaspoon garlic powder
1 teaspoon onion powder
1 teaspoon paprika
  Salt and pepper
4 tablespoons peanut oil

Pepper Relish:

3 medium bell peppers (one each—red, yellow, green), seeded and finely chopped
1 medium red (Bermuda) onion, finely chopped
¼ cup finely chopped fresh Italian flat-leaf parsley
2 large cloves garlic, minced
1 tablespoon tiny capers, drained
1 tablespoon extra-virgin olive oil
1 lemon, squeezed, about 4 tablespoons juice
  Salt and pepper

Line a cookie sheet with a double layer of paper towels. Arrange the tofu slices in a single layer on the paper towels. Cover with a double layer of paper towels

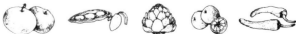

and press lightly to dry the tofu. In a shallow bowl, whisk together the flour, thyme, oregano, red pepper, garlic, onion, paprika, and salt and pepper to taste until well blended. Dredge each tofu slice into the flour mixture, coating both sides evenly. Shake off excess. Set the coated tofu slices onto a large platter or another cookie sheet as you coat them.

Preheat the oven to 350 degrees. Spray a cookie sheet with nonstick cooking spray. Set aside. Heat 2 tablespoons of the peanut oil in a large skillet over medium-high heat. Arrange as many of the tofu slices as you can in a single layer, without crowding. Cook for about 5 minutes, until the tofu slices blacken, then carefully turn the slices over and blacken the other side for about 5 minutes. Transfer to the prepared pan. Heat the remaining 2 tablespoons of peanut oil and cook (blacken) the remaining tofu slices. Transfer the tofu slices to the pan with the other tofu slices. Bake for 20 minutes.

Meanwhile, prepare the pepper relish: Combine all the ingredients in a bowl. Toss well to combine. Taste for seasonings. Remove the tofu slices from the oven and arrange them on a serving platter. Spoon a little of the pepper relish and its juices on the center of each slice.

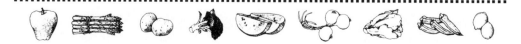

Tofu and Broccoli Divan

SERVES 6

Over the years, I have often heard my friend Louise Povinelli talk about her family's favorite dish: chicken divan. Her vivid description of this treat inspired me to make a vegetarian version under her careful supervision. It's no wonder her family raves over the dish—you'll want to drink the sauce, but don't: Save it for the noodles.

 2 pounds firm tofu, drained and cut into ¼-inch slices lengthwise
 ¼ cup plus 3 tablespoons flour
 2 teaspoons dried sage
   Salt and pepper
 1 large bunch broccoli, florets finely chopped, stems trimmed and saved for
   another use
 3 tablespoons soybean margarine (found in health food stores) or
   canola oil
 1 large shallot, minced
 1 small sweet onion, minced
 ½ cup sweet sherry
 2 cups soy milk (found in supermarkets and health food stores)
 ¼ teaspoon nutmeg
 1 lemon, squeezed, about 2½ tablespoons juice
 1 cup dairy-free mayonnaise (found in health food stores)
 ½ cup plain dry bread crumbs
 1 cup shredded Cheddar or soy cheese (optional)
12 ounces wide noodles, cooked according to package directions

Line a cookie sheet with a double layer of paper towels. Arrange the tofu slices in a single layer over the paper towels. Cover with another double layer of paper towels. Gently press the tofu slices to dry them. In a shallow bowl, whisk together ¼ cup of the flour, 1 teaspoon of the sage, and a little salt and pepper to combine. Spray a large baking pan (large enough to hold the tofu slices in a single layer) with nonstick cooking spray. Dredge the tofu slices in the flour mixture, coating both sides. Shake off excess. Arrange the tofu slices in a single layer in the

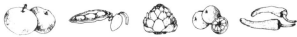

prepared dish. Scatter the broccoli florets evenly over the tofu slices. Sprinkle with salt and pepper.

Preheat the oven to 350 degrees. Melt the soy margarine or heat the oil in a large deep skillet over medium heat. Add the shallot and onion. Cover and cook for 5 minutes, stirring occasionally, until the shallot softens. Whisk in the remaining 3 tablespoons of the flour. Stir constantly for about 2 minutes, scraping the pan, until the mixture cooks. Gradually, whisk in the sherry and soy milk, whisking continuously for about 1 minute until the mixture is smooth. Whisk in the remaining 1 teaspoon of the sage, the nutmeg, lemon juice, mayonnaise, and salt and pepper to taste, whisking until smooth. Continue cooking, uncovered, for 2 minutes, stirring constantly, until the sauce thickens slightly. Taste for seasonings.

Pour the sauce evenly over the broccoli and tofu slices. Sprinkle the bread crumbs evenly over the sauce. Scatter the Cheddar cheese (if using) evenly over the bread crumbs. Cover tightly with foil. Bake for about 1 hour, or until the broccoli is just tender when pierced with a fork. Arrange the cooked noodles on a large serving platter. Spoon the Tofu and Broccoli Divan evenly over the top.

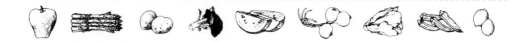

Zucchini in Curry Sauce with Rice and Golden Raisins

SERVES 6

*At **Claire's**, we have discovered that curry enhances the flavors of many vegetables. Zucchini is a delicious example.*

- 3 tablespoons soybean margarine (found in health food stores)
- 2 medium yellow onions, coarsely chopped
- 5 medium zucchini, cut into ¼-inch slices
- 1 tablespoon curry powder or to taste
- ⅛ teaspoon ground red pepper (cayenne)
- ¼ cup mango chutney (found in the condiment section of supermarkets)
- 1 bay leaf
- ½ cup orange juice
- ½ cup golden raisins
  Salt and pepper
- 3 cups cooked jasmine or basmati rice
- 1 cup soy milk

Melt the margarine in a large deep skillet over medium heat. Add the onions and zucchini. Sprinkle with the curry powder and the ground red pepper. Cover and cook for 15 minutes, stirring occasionally, until the vegetables are softened and have released some of their liquids. Stir in the chutney, bay leaf, orange juice, raisins, and salt and pepper to taste. Cover and continue cooking for about 10 minutes, stirring occasionally, until the vegetables are tender. Remove the bay leaf. Stir in the cooked rice. Stir in the soy milk, stirring until well mixed and heated through. Taste for seasonings.

    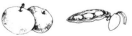

Tofu with Mushrooms Marsala

SERVES 6

This is my adaptation of chicken marsala, a classic Italian dish made with robustly sweet marsala wine. Serve this delicious dish with Scalloped Potatoes (page 106) and Asparagus with Warm Mustard Vinaigrette (page 84) for an elegant meal.

    2 pounds firm tofu, drained
    ¼ cup flour
       Salt and pepper
    3 tablespoons soybean margarine (found in health food stores) or canola oil
    2 large shallots, minced
    1 pound assorted mushrooms, cut into ¼-inch slices
    1 cup marsala wine
    1 tablespoon arrowroot powder or cornstarch

Cut the tofu into ¼-inch slices, lengthwise. Gently pat the slices dry using a double thickness of paper towels. In a shallow bowl, whisk together the flour, and salt and pepper to taste. Dredge the tofu "cutlets" into the flour, coating both sides. Shake off excess. Set the cutlets on a cookie sheet.

Melt the margarine or heat the oil in a large nonstick skillet over medium heat. Add the shallots. Cook for 5 minutes, stirring occasionally, until they are softened. Arrange as many tofu cutlets as you can fit into the skillet without crowding. Cook each side for 3 minutes until golden brown, turning gently to brown the other side. Transfer the tofu cutlets to a cookie sheet. Continue browning the remaining tofu cutlets. Add the mushrooms to the skillet. Sprinkle with salt and pepper. Cover and cook for 5 to 8 minutes, stirring and scraping the bottom of the skillet using a wooden spoon, until the mushrooms are just tender.

Return the tofu cutlets to the skillet, arranging them in a single layer over the mushrooms. Pour ¾ of a cup of the marsala evenly over the tofu and mushrooms. Raise the heat to medium-high. Cover and cook for 15 minutes, moving the pan in a circular motion to mix. In a small bowl, whisk together the remaining ¼ cup marsala and the arrowroot, whisking until smooth. Pour this over the cutlets, moving the pan in a circular motion, and stirring with a plastic spatula to mix evenly. Cook for 1 to 2 minutes, stirring frequently, until the mixture has thickened. Taste for seasonings.

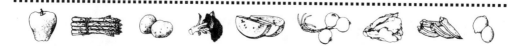

Maryland-Style Tofu Cakes

MAKES 8 CAKES

If you've ever visited Maryland, then you know of its legendary crab cakes. Serve these delicious "crab" cakes to anyone who tells you they don't like tofu. And serve them to anyone who loves tofu and, of course, to everyone who loves crab cakes. They are that good. Serve the tofu cakes with lemon wedges, cocktail sauce, or dairy-free tartar sauce (see Note).

1½ pounds soft tofu, drained
3 tablespoons extra-virgin olive oil
1 lemon, squeezed, about 3 tablespoons juice
2 tablespoons spicy brown mustard
2 tablespoons dairy-free mayonnaise (found in health food stores) or low-fat mayonnaise
¼ cup finely chopped fresh Italian flat-leaf parsley
½ teaspoon dried thyme
½ teaspoon Old Bay seasoning
Salt and pepper
¼ cup minced red (Bermuda) onion
2½ cups plain dry bread crumbs

Place the tofu, 2 tablespoons of the olive oil, lemon juice, mustard, mayonnaise, parsley, thyme, and Old Bay seasoning in a blender. Sprinkle with salt and pepper to taste. Cover and blend on high for 30 seconds, until smooth, stopping every 5 to 10 seconds to scrape down the sides using a rubber spatula. Turn this mixture into a bowl, using the rubber spatula to scrape all of the mixture from the blender. Add the onion, and 2 cups of the bread crumbs. Stir well to combine. Taste for seasonings.

Measure the remaining ½ cup of bread crumbs into a shallow bowl. Using about ½ cup of the tofu mixture per patty, form the tofu mixture into 8 round cakes, using your hands to shape. Carefully (the mixture will be soft), use two hands to coat both sides of the tofu cakes with the bread crumbs. Transfer the coated tofu cakes to a nonstick cookie sheet.

Preheat the oven to 350 degrees. Heat a large nonstick skillet over medium-

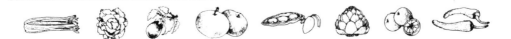

high heat. Brush the skillet generously with about 1½ tablespoons of the remaining olive oil. Carefully arrange the tofu cakes in a single layer in the skillet, without overcrowding. Cook the tofu cakes for 2 to 3 minutes until golden brown. Carefully turn each tofu cake over and cook the other side for another 2 to 3 minutes until golden brown. Return the browned tofu cakes to the nonstick cookie sheet. Repeat the process with the remaining tofu cakes, adding more oil as needed and transferring the browned tofu cakes to the nonstick cookie sheet. After all of the tofu cakes are browned, place the cookie sheet in the oven. Bake for 20 minutes, then carefully turn each tofu cake over and bake the other side for another 20 minutes until heated through when tested with a fork gently inserted in the center of a tofu cake. The tines of the fork will feel hot when the tofu cakes are sufficiently heated. Serve hot.

NOTE: Prepare a dairy-free tartar sauce by simply mixing about ¾ cup of dairy-free mayonnaise with ⅓ cup of pickle relish and a few finely chopped capers.

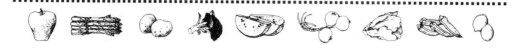

Tofu Cutlets Veracruz-Style

SERVES 6

Serve this delicious dish of tofu cooked in a traditional Mexican sauce of tomatoes, Spanish olives, and onions, with Southwestern Black Bean Salad with Chipotle-Lime Dressing (page 42), corn tortillas, and Mexican Vegetables and Pinto Beans over Yellow Rice (page 238) for a luscious, satisfying meal.

2 pounds firm tofu, drained and cut into ¼-inch slices lengthwise
¼ cup flour
3 tablespoons olive oil
3 large cloves garlic, minced
2 medium sweet onions, coarsely chopped
1 jalapeño pepper, chopped (wash your hands immediately after handling the hot pepper)
½ cup coarsely chopped fresh cilantro
½ cup coarsely chopped, pimento-stuffed Spanish olives, drained
1 28-ounce can Italian whole peeled tomatoes, with juice, squeezed with your hands to crush
Salt and pepper

Drain the excess water from the sliced tofu cutlets on a cookie sheet lined with a double layer of paper towels. Place a double layer of paper towels on top of the tofu slices, and gently pat dry. Measure the flour into a shallow bowl. Dredge the tofu slices in the flour, coating both sides. Shake off excess. Heat the olive oil in a large deep skillet over medium heat. Brown each side of the tofu slices for about 3 minutes per side, in two batches. Transfer the browned slices to a platter. Add the garlic, onions, jalapeño pepper, cilantro, and Spanish olives to the skillet. Cover and cook for 5 minutes, stirring occasionally, until the onions have released some of their liquids. Add the tomatoes and salt and pepper to taste. Cover and bring to a boil. Cook at a low-medium boil for about 25 minutes, stirring occasionally.

Return the tofu slices to the skillet, overlapping the slices and spooning the sauce over them. Cover and cook for 10 minutes, occasionally moving the pan in a circular motion to mix. Taste for seasonings.

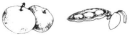

Seitan Osso Buco—Style

SERVES 4

Seitan or "wheat meat" is a meat alternative with the texture of beef, and can be cooked in any dish that normally calls for beef, veal, or chicken. Seitan is made from wheat gluten, and is high in protein and fat-free. You can buy it in small packets in the refrigerated section of health food stores.

- 2 tablespoons extra-virgin olive oil
- 2 tablespoons soybean margarine (found in health food stores) or canola oil
- 4 large cloves garlic, minced
- 1 medium sweet onion, minced
- 1 medium carrot, peeled and minced
- 2 ribs celery with leaves, minced
- 1 12-ounce package seitan, drained, cut into ½-inch slices
- 2 large ripe tomatoes, chopped, including juices
- 1 tablespoon tomato paste
  Salt and pepper
- 1 cup red wine
- 1 bay leaf
- 2 teaspoons dried thyme
- 5 fresh basil leaves, cut in half
- 2 teaspoons finely grated lemon zest
- ¼ finely chopped fresh Italian flat-leaf parsley
- 1 pound potato gnocchi (found in the freezer section of Italian markets and many supermarkets)

Heat the olive oil and margarine in a large deep skillet over medium heat. Add the garlic, onion, carrot, and celery. Cover and cook for 15 minutes, stirring occasionally, until the vegetables have released some of their juices. Add the seitan, tomatoes, tomato paste, salt and pepper to taste, the red wine, bay leaf, thyme, basil, lemon zest, and parsley. Cover and cook for 30 minutes, stirring occasionally, until the tomatoes have softened enough to look like a sauce. Taste for seasonings. Remove the bay leaf. Meanwhile, cook the gnocchi according to package directions. Drain and turn into a serving bowl. Spoon the seitan and the sauce over the gnocchi.

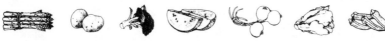

Peppers, Potatoes, and Tofu Hot Dogs

SERVES 6

My mother never made grilled hot dogs for summer cookouts. Instead, she always prepared a flavorful dish of hot dogs with peppers and potatoes for a picnic. My mom was determined to give us vegetables and plenty of them with our meals. Here is my delicious and healthy remake of this memorable dish. It also makes a terrific sandwich filling. For the hot dogs, I like LightLife brand Tofu Pups.

6 medium potatoes, peeled and cut into 1-inch cubes
3 tablespoons extra-virgin olive oil
1 large onion, cut in half lengthwise, then sliced into ½-inch ribs
5 bell peppers (red, yellow, and/or green), cut in half, seeded, then cut into 1-inch pieces
Salt and pepper
1 12-ounce package tofu hot dogs, cut into ½-inch pieces
⅓ cup cooking liquid from the potatoes

Cook the potatoes in lightly salted boiling water for about 10 minutes until crisp-tender. Reserve ⅓ cup of the cooking liquid and set aside. Drain the potatoes and set aside. Heat the olive oil in a large skillet over medium heat. Add the onion and peppers. Sprinkle with salt and pepper to taste. Cover and cook for 20 minutes, stirring occasionally, until crisp-tender. Add the tofu hot dogs. Cover and cook for 5 minutes, stirring occasionally. Add the cooked potatoes and the reserved cooking liquid. Continue cooking, covered, for 3 minutes, stirring occasionally. Taste for seasonings.

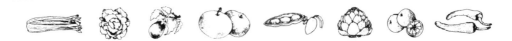

Tofu Hot Dogs Italian-Style, with Red Peppers, Onions, and Tomatoes

SERVES 4

Every Italian mother I know has made her own version of this recipe for a picnic or for supper at one time or another. All the kids I knew growing up looked forward to it, including me. We ate this flavorful combination with Italian bread—either on the side or as a sandwich with this wonderful filling. With the new, extensive variety of "healthy" hot dogs, available either from a health food store or at many supermarkets, you can serve hot dogs with a clear conscience.

1 tablespoon olive oil
4 tofu hot dogs, cut into ½-inch pieces
2 medium sweet onions (Vidalia would be great), cut in half lengthwise, then sliced into ½-inch ribs, separated
3 large red bell peppers, cut in half, seeded, and sliced into 1-inch ribs
  Salt and pepper
½ cup water
2 tablespoons tomato paste

Heat a large nonstick skillet over medium heat. Add the olive oil and tilt the pan to coat the bottom of the skillet. Add the hot dogs. Cover and cook for 2 minutes, stirring occasionally, until lightly browned. Using a slotted plastic spatula, transfer the hot dogs to a plate. Set aside. Add the onions and peppers to the skillet. Sprinkle lightly with salt and pepper. Cover the skillet and cook over medium heat for 30 to 35 minutes, stirring occasionally, until the peppers and onions are soft-tender.

Combine the water and the tomato paste in a cup. Whisk well with a fork to combine. Stir into the pepper and onion mixture in the skillet. Return the hot dogs to the skillet. Stir well to mix together. Cover and continue cooking at a low-medium boil for 5 minutes, stirring occasionally to blend. Taste for seasonings.

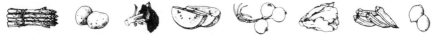

Acorn Squash Stuffed with Cornbread, Rice, Pears, Cranberries, and Pecans

SERVES 4

Stuffed acorn squash is my traditional Thanksgiving entree. We all look forward to enjoying it with Garlic Mashed Potatoes (page 105), Portobello and Cremini Mushroom and Herb Gravy (page 123), Candied Sweet Potatoes (page 108), Cranberry-Lime Sauce (page 124), and a tossed green salad. But why wait until Thanksgiving?

2½ cups water
½ stick (4 tablespoons) soybean margarine (found in health food stores) or canola oil
1 small carrot, peeled and finely chopped
1 rib celery (with leaves), finely chopped
1 small zucchini, finely chopped
Fresh corn kernels cut from 1 large ear of corn (about ¾ cup), *or* frozen kernels
1 pear, cored and coarsely chopped
¼ cup dried or fresh cranberries
Salt and pepper
3 cups cornbread stuffing cubes (found in supermarkets)
1 cup cooked brown rice
1 tablespoon grated orange zest
2 tablespoons chopped pecans
1 tablespoon peeled and grated fresh gingerroot or ½ teaspoon ground ginger
2 large acorn squash, cut in half and seeded

Preheat the oven to 450 degrees. Bring the water and the margarine to a boil in a large covered pot over high heat. Stir in the carrot, celery, zucchini, corn kernels, pear, and cranberries. Sprinkle with salt and pepper. Cover, lower the heat

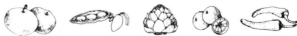

to medium, and cook for 2 minutes, stirring once. Remove from the heat. Stir in the stuffing cubes. Stir well to mix. Add the rice, orange zest, pecans, and ginger. Stir well to mix. Taste for seasonings.

Spray a large roasting pan with nonstick cooking spray. Divide the stuffing among the 4 acorn squash halves, mounding each. Arrange the stuffed halves in the roasting pan, leaving a little space in between each for even roasting. Pour 2 cups of hot water into the pan around, not over, the stuffed squash. Cover the pan with foil, tenting it to avoid touching the stuffing. Bake for about 1¼ hours or until the squash is tender when pierced with a fork.

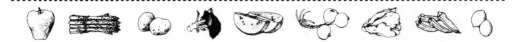

Sicilian Stuffed Eggplant Halves

SERVES 4

My brothers and I often teased our mother about "stuffing everything in sight," which seems to be the Italian way with vegetables. Now I find myself doing the same thing—and loving every mouthful.

- 2 large eggplants, cut in half lengthwise
- 4 tablespoons extra-virgin olive oil
  Salt
- 1 small sweet onion, finely chopped
- 5 large cloves garlic, minced
- ¼ cup golden raisins
- ¼ cup pine nuts
  Pepper
- 2 tablespoons tiny capers, drained
- ¼ cup finely chopped fresh Italian flat-leaf parsley
- 2 teaspoons dried oregano
- 6 cups cooked arborio rice (found in the rice or Italian section of supermarkets)
- ½ cup plain dry bread crumbs, preferably homemade
- 1 28-ounce can Italian whole peeled tomatoes, with juice, squeezed with your hands to crush
- 5 large fresh basil leaves
- ¼ cup red wine

Preheat the oven to 425 degrees. Using a spoon, scoop out some flesh from the eggplant, creating a cavity but leaving about ¼ inch around the edges of the eggplant "shell." Coarsely chop the removed eggplant pulp. Brush the eggplant shells, inside and outside, with 1 to 2 teaspoons of the olive oil. Sprinkle the eggplant with salt. Heat 2½ tablespoons of the olive oil in a large deep skillet over medium heat. Add the chopped eggplant pulp, onion, about half of the minced garlic, the raisins, and pine nuts. Sprinkle with salt and pepper. Cover and cook for 5 minutes, stirring occasionally, until the onions have released some of their liquid. Add the capers, parsley, 1 teaspoon of the oregano, the rice, and bread

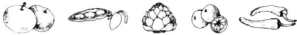

crumbs. Stir well to combine. Taste for seasonings. Divide the stuffing among the eggplant halves.

Spray a large baking pan with nonstick cooking spray. Arrange the eggplant halves in the prepared pan. In a bowl, combine the tomatoes, basil, wine, the remaining 1 tablespoon of olive oil, the remaining garlic, the remaining 1 teaspoon of oregano, and salt and pepper to taste. Stir well to combine. Spoon this sauce over the eggplant halves. Cover tightly with foil. Bake for about 50 minutes until the eggplants are soft-tender when pierced with a fork.

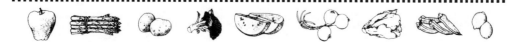

Stuffed Escarole

SERVES 6

My uncle Bob and I were reminiscing about the many wonderful dishes my grandmother in New Haven made, and how you don't see them anymore. Well, I can never resist anything that reminds me of my grandmother, so here is her recipe for special, stuffed escarole. This makes a lovely first course for any Italian meal, but my grandmother would probably serve it to the family as part of dinner, along with a dish of polenta with beans, followed by a huge platter of thin spaghetti in a simple Marinara Sauce (page 178), and a salad tossed with olive oil and fresh lemon juice. A plate of freshly cut fruits, Italian pastries, and espresso would end this typically Amalfitan Sunday meal.

> 1 large head escarole
> 3 cups plain dry bread crumbs, homemade if possible
> 1 rib celery with leaves, minced
> 3 large cloves garlic, minced
> ⅓ cup chopped fresh Italian flat-leaf parsley
> 12 oil-cured black olives, pitted and chopped
> ¼ cup grated Parmesan cheese
> 5 tablespoons extra-virgin olive oil
>   Salt and pepper

Have some twine or heavy thread ready for tying the escarole. Fill your sink with cool water. Hold the head of escarole by the base and thoroughly rinse it by swishing the head back and forth and up and down into the water until all the sand is removed from the leaves all the way down into the base. Spread the leaves with your fingers and look deep into the base where the leaves are white and attached to the base: You'll feel and see any sand or grit that hasn't been rinsed out. After you have thoroughly cleaned the escarole, set it upside down in a colander to drain.

Meanwhile, in a bowl, combine the bread crumbs, celery, garlic, parsley, black olives, and Parmesan cheese. Toss well using two spoons. Drizzle 2 tablespoons of the olive oil evenly over the top. Quickly toss well using two spoons. Taste for salt before adding any, as the Parmesan cheese and the olives may make it salty enough. Add salt and pepper to taste, tossing well to combine.

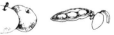

Lift the head of escarole up and set it in a large bowl, with the leaves up and the base down in the bowl. Using your hands, spread the leaves open. Spoon the bread crumb mixture into the center of the escarole. Using your fingers, scatter the bread crumb mixture in between the leaves. Using your hands, gently force the leaves together to form a log-shape bundle. Tie the "bundle" loosely with thread in two to three places to enclose the bread crumb mixture.

Heat the remaining 3 tablespoons of olive oil in a large skillet over medium-low heat. Carefully transfer the escarole to the heated oil, using your hands. Lay it on its side. Cover and cook for 15 minutes, until the leaves are wilted but not browned. Carefully turn the escarole to the other side, using tongs and a plastic spatula. Lower the heat, cover, and continue cooking for about 25 minutes, until the leaves are tender when pierced with a fork. Transfer the escarole to a serving platter. Cut and discard the twine or string. Cut the escarole into 6 serving pieces.

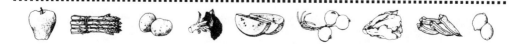

Tempeh and Vegetables in Barbecue Sauce

SERVES 4

Tempeh is a fabulous meat alternative made from fermented soybeans. It has a delicious nutty, light, smoky flavor and it is rich in protein, vitamins, and minerals. You'll love the chewy texture, too. We eat this dish with coleslaw, potato salad, and corn on the cob for a "picnic" any time of year. You can find packages of tempeh (there are several varieties: soy, barley, brown rice, and millet) in the refrigerated or frozen foods sections of many supermarkets and in all health food stores.

2 tablespoons extra-virgin olive oil
1 large sweet onion, cut into ½-inch ribs
1 large green bell pepper, seeded and sliced into ½-inch ribs
8 ounces soy tempeh, chopped into 1-inch cubes
1 pound mushrooms, sliced (button, shiitake, and cremini would be nice, but any variety will be fine)
1 large ripe tomato, chopped
3 tablespoons water
Salt and pepper
½ cup bottled barbecue sauce

Heat the olive oil in a large, nonstick skillet over medium-high heat. Add the onion, pepper, and tempeh. Cover and cook for about 10 minutes, stirring frequently, until the tempeh is lightly browned. Add the mushrooms and tomato. Sprinkle with the water, and salt and pepper to taste. Stir well to mix. Continue cooking, uncovered, for 5 minutes, stirring frequently. Stir in the barbecue sauce. Continue cooking, uncovered, for 5 to 10 minutes, stirring frequently, until the peppers and the mushrooms are as tender as you like and the sauce is thickened slightly. Taste for seasonings.

    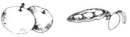

"Sausage"-and-Broccoli-Stuffed Mushroom Caps

SERVES 6

You are in for a wonderful and tasty surprise if you haven't yet tasted mush-rooms stuffed with meatless sausage. I use LightLife Italian Links, found in health food stores. You can also substitute soy mozzarella-style cheese (found at health food stores), or provolone if you prefer a sharp flavor.

12 large mushrooms for stuffing, about 1¾ pounds
 3 tablespoons olive oil
 3 large cloves garlic, minced
 1 teaspoon crushed red pepper
 4 cups finely chopped broccoli florets (from about 2 stalks of broccoli)
 4 links meatless sausage, finely chopped
 Salt and pepper
 5 to 6 large clean arugula leaves, finely chopped
 ¼ cup coarsely shredded low-fat or fat-free mozzarella
 1 egg or equivalent egg substitute, lightly beaten
 ¼ cup plain dry bread crumbs

Preheat the oven to 375 degrees. Remove stems from mushrooms. Reserve the stems for another use (sauce, stuffing, or soup). Briefly rinse and drain the mush-room caps. Arrange the caps cut-side up in a roasting pan large enough to fit the caps in a single layer. Set aside. Heat the oil in a large skillet over a low heat. Add the garlic and crushed red pepper. Cook for 2 minutes, stirring frequently. Add the florets and the sausage. Using a wooden spoon, break up the chopped sausage into little pieces. Add salt and pepper to taste. Cover and cook over low heat for 10 minutes, stirring occasionally, until the broccoli is just tender. Stir in the arugula. Cover and continue cooking for 1 minute, stirring frequently. Remove from heat and turn into a bowl. Add the shredded cheese, egg, and bread crumbs. Stir well to combine. Taste for seasonings.

Fill the mushroom caps, mounding slightly with your hands. Pour 2 cups of water into the pan around, not over, the filled caps. Cover tightly with foil, tenting if needed so that the foil does not touch the stuffing. Bake on the bottom rack for 20 minutes, then remove the foil and continue baking for 10 minutes until brown.

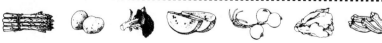

Acorn Squash with Rice and Vegetable Stuffing

SERVES 4

We have always been big fans of acorn squash in my family, thanks in no small part to all of the delicious ways my mom prepared this vitamin-packed vegetable.

3 tablespoons extra-virgin olive oil
1 medium sweet onion, finely chopped
1 cup finely chopped broccoli florets
1 medium carrot, peeled and finely diced
1 medium apple, any variety, finely chopped
5 ounces spinach, washed well and finely chopped
1 medium ripe tomato, finely chopped, including juices
¼ cup coarsely chopped fresh Italian flat-leaf parsley
¼ cup pine nuts
   Salt and pepper
6 cups cooked arborio rice (found in the rice or Italian section of supermarkets)
4 large acorn squash, cut in half, seeded

Preheat the oven to 450 degrees. Heat the olive oil in a large deep skillet over medium heat. Add the onion, broccoli florets, carrot, apple, spinach, tomato, parsley, and pine nuts. Sprinkle with salt and pepper to taste. Cover and cook for about 5 minutes, stirring occasionally, until the vegetables are crisp-tender. Stir in the rice, mixing well to combine. Taste for seasonings. Divide the stuffing among the squash halves, mounding the stuffing. Arrange the filled halves in a large baking pan and pour about 2 cups of water into the pan around, not on, the squash to 1 inch deep. Cover the pan tightly with foil, tenting the foil as needed. Bake for about 1¼ hours, until the squash is fork-tender.

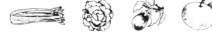

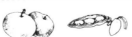

Jumbo Mushroom Caps Filled with Spinach, Tofu, and Sun-Dried Tomatoes

SERVES 4

These savory mushrooms make a lovely presentation for a buffet. You can prepare the stuffing and fill the mushroom caps a day in advance. Serve them with Sweet Cinnamon Carrots (page 93) and Italian Green Bean and Potato Salad (page 62).

1 pound large mushrooms (about 10), stems removed (save for a salad or soup)
8 ounces soft tofu, drained
1 large clove garlic, chopped
2 tablespoons extra-virgin olive oil
2 tablespoons pine nuts
2 tablespoons finely chopped fresh Italian flat-leaf parsley
  Salt and pepper
2 tablespoons minced, sun-dried tomatoes, drained if oil-packed
1 cup minced fresh spinach
1 cup plain dry bread crumbs, preferably homemade
½ lemon, squeezed, about 1 tablespoon juice

Preheat the oven to 400 degrees. Briefly rinse the mushroom caps under cool water. Drain in a colander with the cap-side down. Place the tofu, garlic, olive oil, pine nuts, and parsley in a blender. Sprinkle lightly with salt and pepper. Cover and blend on high speed for about 20 seconds, stopping 4 to 5 times to scrape down the sides using a rubber spatula, until the mixture is blended. Turn the tofu mixture into a bowl. Add the tomatoes, spinach, bread crumbs, and lemon juice. Stir well to mix. Taste for seasonings.

Spoon the stuffing into the mushroom caps, using your hands to mound the filling. Arrange the mushrooms in a baking pan. Pour 1 cup of hot water into the baking pan around, not over, the mushrooms. Cover tightly with foil, tenting it as needed to avoid touching the filling. Bake for 45 minutes. Remove the foil and continue baking for another 10 minutes or until the mushrooms are tender when pierced with a fork and the filling is golden brown.

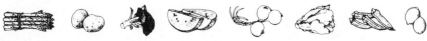

Artichoke Pie

SERVES 6

This is a great Italian pie to serve at a cocktail party and it makes a lovely, light dinner when served with a salad and bread.

- 3 tablespoons extra-virgin olive oil
- 1 medium sweet onion, finely chopped
- 1 large clove garlic, minced
- ¼ cup finely chopped fresh Italian flat-leaf parsley
- 1 11 ounce can artichoke hearts, drained and chopped
- 6 eggs or egg substitute, lightly beaten
- 5 large basil leaves, finely chopped
- 1 cup shredded mozzarella cheese or soy cheese (found in health food stores)
- 3 tablespoons grated Parmesan cheese or soy cheese (found in health food stores)
  Salt and pepper
- 1 9-inch unbaked pie crust (store bought is fine)

Preheat oven to 350 degrees. Heat the olive oil in a skillet over medium heat. Add the onions, garlic, and parsley. Cook for 5 minutes, stirring occasionally, until the onions have softened. Remove from heat and turn into a bowl, using a rubber spatula to scrape the pan. Stir in the artichoke hearts, eggs, basil leaves, mozzarella, Parmesan, and salt and pepper to taste. Stir to mix well. Place the pie pan on a cookie sheet to catch any drippings. Pour the artichoke mixture into the pie shell, using a rubber spatula to scrape the bowl. Bake the pie for about 40 minutes or until the center is set and the crust is golden brown. Allow to set for 10 minutes before serving.

    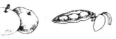

Stuffed Pepper Halves

SERVES 6

My mother-in-law is one of my favorite cooks. This is her recipe for the best stuffed peppers in the world.

- 1 12-ounce loaf day-old Italian or French bread
- 4 cups warm water
- 6 bell peppers (red, green, and/or yellow)
- 5 large cloves garlic, finely chopped
- ¼ cup finely chopped fresh Italian flat-leaf parsley
- 1 medium zucchini, cut into ¼-inch dice
- 6 large mushrooms (button and shiitake), thinly sliced
- 1 small onion, minced
- 3 tablespoons extra-virgin olive oil
- 1 teaspoon dried oregano
- Salt and pepper
- 1 egg or egg substitute, lightly beaten
- 1 cup hot water

Preheat the oven to 400 degrees. Cut the bread into 10 pieces. Place the bread in a large bowl. Pour 4 cups of warm water over the bread. Using your hand, push the bread to the bottom of the bowl so the bread will soften as it absorbs the warm water. Set the bread aside for 5 minutes. Drain the bread in a colander. Squeeze out as much water as you can, using your hand, pushing down on the bread into the colander. Turn the drained bread into a large bowl.

Cut ¼ inch off the top of each pepper. Mince the top pieces (discard the stems) and add them to the bread. Cut each pepper in half. Remove and discard the seeds and the soft ribs from each pepper half. Set aside. Add the garlic, parsley, zucchini, mushrooms, and onion to the bread. Toss well to mix. Drizzle the olive oil over the bread mixture. Add the oregano, and salt and pepper to taste. Add the egg. Toss well to combine.

Divide the filling among the pepper halves, mounding as necessary. Place the pepper halves in a large roasting pan. Pour the hot water around, not over, the peppers. Cover tightly with foil. Bake for 45 to 60 minutes until the peppers are fork-tender.

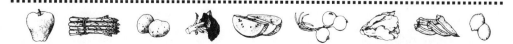

Spinach, Tomato, and Goat Cheese Pizzas

SERVES 6

Thick Greek pita breads make excellent pizzas, and they are so convenient. I keep them in my freezer and defrost (they defrost in no time) six at a time for this delicious and easy entree. I like to serve these pizzas for dinner with Basmati Rice with Green Peas and Pine Nuts (page 119), and corn on the cob.

6 7 to 8 inch Greek pita breads
3 tablespoons extra-virgin olive oil
5 large cloves garlic, chopped
2 large ripe tomatoes, finely chopped
   Salt and pepper
2 10-ounce bags spinach, well washed and chopped
5 to 6 ounces goat cheese, crumbled

Preheat the oven to 350 degrees. Arrange the pita breads in a single layer on nonstick cookie sheets (or spray cookie sheets with cooking oil). Set aside. Heat the olive oil in a large skillet over a low-medium heat. Add the garlic and cook for 3 to 4 minutes, stirring occasionally, until softened. Stir in the tomatoes. Sprinkle with salt and pepper. Continue cooking for 3 to 4 minutes, stirring occasionally, until they begin to release their liquid. Add the spinach. Cover and cook for about 5 minutes, stirring occasionally, until the spinach is wilted. Taste for seasonings. Using a slotted spoon, spread the spinach and tomato mixture evenly over the pita breads. Scatter the goat cheese evenly over the pizzas. Bake for about 10 to 12 minutes until the goat cheese melts slightly. Serve immediately.

Mushroom Quesadillas

SERVES 6

Quesadillas are like Mexican grilled cheese sandwiches, and they are just as easy to prepare. Serve these quesadillas with Maple-Glazed, Apple-Stuffed Acorn Squash (page 99) and Refried Black Beans (page 113) or Mexican Vegetables and Pinto Beans over Yellow Rice (page 238).

>   2 tablespoons plus 1 teaspoon olive oil
>   2 medium onions, coarsely chopped
>   2 scallions, white part and 4 inches of green, coarsely chopped
>   5 ounces spinach, well washed and coarsely chopped
>   1 pound mixed button and cremini mushrooms, cut into ¼-inch slices
>   ¼ cup coarsely chopped fresh cilantro
>   2 teaspoons chili powder
>   1 teaspoon cumin
>   Salt and pepper
>   10 8-inch flour tortillas
>   2 cups shredded Monterey Jack cheese

Heat 2 tablespoons of the olive oil in a large skillet over medium heat. Add the onions, scallions, spinach, mushrooms, and cilantro. Cover and cook for 25 minutes, stirring occasionally until the mushrooms are tender. Sprinkle the chili powder, cumin, and salt and pepper to taste, evenly over the vegetables. Stir well to combine. Continue cooking, uncovered, for 1 minute, stirring occasionally. Taste for seasonings.

Preheat the oven to 350 degrees. Arrange 4 tortillas in a single layer on two nonstick cookie sheets or on two cookie sheets sprayed with nonstick cooking spray. Scatter about 3 tablespoons of shredded cheese evenly over each of the tortillas. Using a slotted spoon, transfer one fourth of the mushroom mixture to each of the tortillas. Scatter the remaining shredded cheese evenly over the vegetables. Top with the remaining 4 tortillas, pressing down. Brush the tops of the tortillas evenly with the remaining 1 teaspoon of olive oil. Bake the quesadillas for 10 minutes or until just golden brown. Remove from oven. Cut each quesadilla into quarters. Serve immediately.

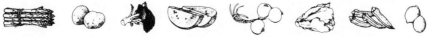

Mexican Vegetables and Pinto Beans over Yellow Rice

SERVES 8

Pinto beans, along with other traditional Mexican ingredients, have certainly grown in popularity and in availability over the years. Top this dish with sour cream and some finely chopped raw onion or sliced avocado.

  3 tablespoons olive oil
  2 medium sweet onions, coarsely chopped
  3 quarts water
 12 ounces pinto beans, picked over for stones (about 1¾ cups)
 ¼ cup finely chopped fresh cilantro or parsley
  3 medium carrots, peeled and cut into ½-inch slices
  2 teaspoons ground cumin
  2 teaspoons chili powder
  2 medium zucchini, cut into ½-inch slices
  4 scallions, white part and 3 inches of green, coarsely chopped
    Fresh corn kernels cut from 3 large ears corn (about 3 cups), *or*
    2 10-ounce packages frozen kernels
    Salt and pepper

Yellow Rice:

3¾ cups water
1½ cups brown rice
  2 tablespoons annatto seed (anchiote—found in the spice section or the Latin section of most supermarkets)
    Salt and pepper

Heat the olive oil in a large soup pot over medium heat. Add the onions. Cook for 5 minutes, stirring occasionally, until the onions are softened. Add 3 quarts of water and the pinto beans. Cover and raise the heat to high. Bring to a boil, then lower the heat to medium. Cook, covered, at a medium boil for 45 minutes, stirring occasionally. Add the cilantro, carrots, cumin, and chili powder. Cook, uncovered, for about 45 minutes, stirring occasionally, until the beans are just tender. Stir in zucchini, scallions, and salt and pepper to taste. Cook for 30 minutes, stirring occasionally. Stir in the corn. Cook for 5 minutes, stirring occasionally.

Meanwhile, prepare the yellow rice: Put 3¾ cups water and the rice into a 3-quart pot. Wrap the annatto seeds in cheesecloth and tie it in a knot to secure, or use a teaball to hold the seeds. Place the wrapped seeds in the pot with the rice and water. Cover and place over high heat. Bring to a boil, then lower the heat to low and cook at a low boil for about 40 minutes, stirring occasionally, until the rice is tender and the water is absorbed. Remove and discard the annatto seeds. Stir in salt and pepper to taste. Remove from heat and keep covered until the vegetables and pinto beans are cooked. Serve over the yellow rice.

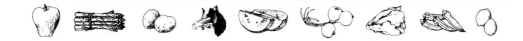

Sweet and White Potato Burritos with Avocado-Jalapeño Sauce

SERVES 6

This Mexican dish is a favorite in my house. I serve the filling in a bowl, with the tortillas and the sauce on the side. Everyone makes their own burritos or enjoys the elements separately, eating the tortilla as they would any other bread. I wrote this recipe with the sensitive palate in mind, but you can certainly increase the fire by adding additional cayenne pepper to the filling. Serve these wonderful burritos with Refried Black Beans (page 113) and Fresh Corn Salad with Chipotle Vinaigrette (page 45).

- 3 large sweet potatoes, peeled and cut into 1-inch chunks
- 3 medium white potatoes, peeled and cut into 1-inch chunks
- 3 tablespoons peanut oil
- 1 large onion, chopped
- ¼ cup chopped fresh cilantro
  Salt and pepper
- 1 teaspoon chili powder
- ¼ teaspoon ground red pepper (cayenne)
- ½ teaspoon dried oregano
- 6 10-inch flour tortillas

Avocado-Jalapeño Sauce:

- 1 medium avocado
- 1 small onion, chopped
- 1 small jalapeño pepper, seeded and chopped (wash your hands immediately after handling hot peppers)
- ¼ cup coarsely chopped fresh cilantro
- 2 cups (16 ounces) low-fat or fat-free sour cream
  Salt and pepper

Cook the white and sweet potatoes in lightly salted, boiling water for about 10 minutes, until they are not quite tender. Reserve ⅓ cup of cooking liquid and set aside. Drain the potatoes. Heat the peanut oil in a large skillet over low-medium heat. Add the onion. Cook for 4 to 5 minutes, stirring occasionally, until softened. Add the cilantro and the cooked potatoes. Sprinkle with salt and pepper to taste, the chili powder, cayenne, and oregano. Add the reserved ⅓ cup cooking liquid. Raise the heat to medium. Continue cooking, uncovered, for about 5 minutes, until the potatoes are tender, stirring occasionally. Taste for seasonings. Lower heat to warm. Cover and keep warm while you prepare the sauce.

Cut the avocado in half lengthwise. Separate the halves by twisting them apart. Scoop out and discard the pit with a spoon. Scoop out the avocado pulp with a spoon, scraping as close to the skin as possible. Place the avocado pulp in a blender. Place the remaining sauce ingredients into the blender. Cover. Blend on high speed for 3 seconds. Stop and scrape down the sides, using a rubber spatula. Cover and continue blending on high speed for 10 to 12 seconds, stopping 3 or 4 times to scrape down the sides, until the sauce is smooth. Taste for seasonings.

To assemble the burritos: Lay one tortilla on a dinner plate. Spread about one sixth of the filling in a line down the center of the tortilla. Lift each side of the tortilla over the filling, covering the filling. Carefully turn the tortilla over, so that the seam side is down. Spoon about ½ cup of the sauce over the tortilla. Repeat until all the burritos are prepared. Serve immediately.

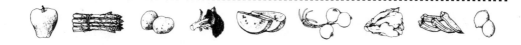

Black Bean Quesadillas

SERVES 6

*We love black beans at my house and at **Claire's**. They are not only delicious in these quesadillas but are also rich in iron, calcium, and protein. I like to cook the beans the night before I plan to make the quesadillas. This gives me a delicious and quick dinner for those busy weeknights when time is so limited. Serve them with Avocado, Tomato, and Onion Salad (page 33); they are perfectly delicious together.*

12 ounces black beans, cooked according to package directions
 2 tablespoons plus 1 teaspoon olive oil
 1 medium zucchini, finely diced
 2 medium cloves garlic, minced
 1 teaspoon chili powder
    Salt and pepper
10 8-inch flour tortillas
 8 ounces shredded low-fat Monterey Jack cheese
 1 cup fat-free sour cream (optional)

Preheat the oven to 350 degrees. Drain the black beans and set them aside. Heat 2 tablespoons of the olive oil in a large skillet over medium heat. Add the zucchini and the garlic. Stir in the chili powder and sprinkle with salt and pepper to taste. Cover and cook for 10 minutes, stirring occasionally until tender. Remove from the heat. Stir in the cooked black beans. Taste for seasonings.

Spray 2 cookie sheets with nonstick cooking spray. Arrange 2 flour tortillas in a single layer on each cookie sheet. Sprinkle half of the cheese evenly over the tortillas. Spoon one quarter (about 1 cup) of the black bean filling evenly over each of the four tortillas. Sprinkle the remaining cheese evenly over the beans. Cover each tortilla with one of the remaining tortillas. Press down lightly on the tortillas, using your hand. Brush the tops of the tortillas with the remaining teaspoon of olive oil. Bake on the top rack for 10 minutes until the tortillas are golden brown. Cut each quesadilla into quarters before serving with a dollop of sour cream, if desired.

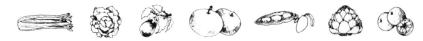

Spinach Pie

SERVES 6

This pie of fresh spinach and ricotta cheese with a little sausage makes a delicious Italian dinner. Serve it with Fresh Tomato Salad (page 54) and Italian-Style Sautéed Cauliflower (page 94).

- 3 tablespoons extra-virgin olive oil
- 1 medium sweet onion, finely chopped
- 5 ounces meatless Italian sausage (LightLife Foods makes Lean Links, found at health food stores), cut into ¼-inch pieces
- 1 large clove garlic, minced
- 2 10-ounce bags spinach, washed well and coarsely chopped
  Salt and pepper
- ½ cup ricotta cheese
- 3 eggs or equivalent egg substitute, lightly beaten
- 4 ounces shredded mozzarella cheese (about 1 cup)
- 2 tablespoons grated Romano cheese
- 1 9-inch unbaked pie crust (store bought is fine)

Heat the olive oil in a large deep skillet over medium heat. Add the onion, sausage, and garlic. Cover and cook for 10 minutes, stirring occasionally, until the onions and sausage are lightly browned. Using a slotted spoon, transfer the onions, garlic, and sausage to a bowl. Add the spinach to the skillet. Sprinkle with salt and pepper. Cover and cook for 10 minutes, stirring occasionally, until the spinach is wilted.

Preheat the oven to 350 degrees. Drain the spinach in a colander and add to the onion mixture. Add the ricotta cheese, eggs, mozzarella, and Romano cheese. Stir well to mix thoroughly. Place the pie crust on a cookie sheet. Turn the filling into the pie crust, using a rubber spatula to scrape the bowl. Bake the pie for about 40 minutes or until the center is set. Remove from the oven and allow the pie to set for 10 minutes before cutting into 6 serving pieces.

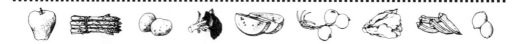

Shepherd's Pie

SERVES 4

Who could resist such a tasty vegetarian rendition of this old favorite? This one-dish meal of vegetable burgers, spinach, corn, and mashed potatoes needs only a tossed salad to make a wonderful dinner.

- 4 meatless burgers, partially defrosted and cut in half (see Note)
- 2 tablespoons olive oil
- 1 10-ounce bag of spinach, thoroughly rinsed and well drained, coarsely chopped
  Salt and pepper
  Fresh corn kernels cut from 2 large ears of corn (about 1½ cups), *or*
  1 10-ounce package frozen kernels
- 3 cups cooked mashed potatoes (from about 5 large potatoes)
- 3 tablespoons plain bread crumbs (fresh, if possible)
- 2 tablespoons freshly grated Romano cheese (optional)

Preheat oven to 400 degrees. Spray a large rectangular baking dish with nonstick cooking spray. Arrange the halved vegetable burgers to fit in a single layer on the bottom of the baking dish. Set aside. Heat the olive oil in a large, nonstick skillet over a low-medium heat. Add the chopped spinach. Don't worry if the spinach is mounded high in the skillet; it will shrink down as it cooks. Sprinkle with salt and pepper to taste. Cover (or set the cover on top of the mound of spinach) and cook for about 7 minutes, turning occasionally, using tongs, until the spinach is wilted. Stir in the corn kernels. Cover and continue cooking for 3 minutes, stirring occasionally. Taste for seasonings. Spoon this mixture evenly over the vegetable burgers. Spoon the mashed potatoes on top, using the back of the spoon to smooth them across the top. Sprinkle evenly with the bread crumbs and the Romano cheese, if using. Bake for 40 minutes, until the vegetable burgers are cooked and the potatoes are heated through when tested with a fork. Use a metal spatula for serving.

NOTE: Most supermarkets (and all health food stores) carry at least one brand of meatless burgers in their frozen food section. I like Morning Star Farms, LightLife Foods, Green Giant's Harvest Burgers, and Boca Burgers brands best, but try a variety and decide on your favorite brand.

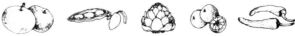

Sicilian Rice Balls

SERVES 8

I like to serve these with warm Marinara Sauce (page 178) for dipping. Bite-size rice balls make lovely appetizers for a cocktail party.

- 5 cups water
- 1 pound arborio rice (found in the rice or the Italian section of supermarkets)
- 1 cup shredded mozzarella cheese
- ¼ cup grated Parmesan cheese
- ½ cup minced fresh Italian flat-leaf parsley
  Salt and pepper
- 4 eggs or equivalent egg substitute, lightly beaten
- 3 cups plain dry bread crumbs
- ½ cup olive oil

Bring the water to a boil in a covered pot over high heat. Stir in the rice. Lower the heat to low. Cover and cook the rice for about 25 minutes, stirring frequently, until the water is absorbed and the rice is tender. Remove from the heat. Turn the rice into a bowl. Stir in the mozzarella, Parmesan, and parsley, mixing well to melt the mozzarella. Add salt and pepper to taste. Cover and refrigerate for at least an hour until cool enough to handle.

Scoop ¼ cupful of the rice mixture into your hand and roll into a ball. Set the rice ball on a cookie sheet. Continue forming all of the rice mixture into (24) balls. In a shallow bowl, beat the eggs lightly. Measure the bread crumbs into a separate shallow bowl. Roll each rice ball into the beaten eggs to coat, then lift out and shake off excess. Roll the rice ball in the bread crumbs to coat. Shake off excess. Place the breaded rice balls back onto the cookie sheet, and repeat with the remaining rice balls until they are all breaded.

Preheat the oven to 350 degrees. Spray a separate cookie sheet with nonstick cooking spray. Set aside. Heat ¼ cup of the olive oil in a large skillet over medium-high heat. Place as many rice balls into the heated oil as you can fit without crowding. Brown the rice balls evenly on all sides, cooking 1 to 2 minutes per side, until evenly browned. Transfer the browned rice balls to the prepared cookie sheet. Heat the remaining ¼ cup olive oil. Continue browning the remaining rice balls. Bake the rice balls for 20 minutes to heat through. Serve alone or with lemon wedges or warm Marinara Sauce.

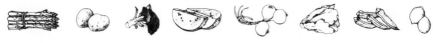

Broccoli Rabe with White Beans and Potatoes

SERVES 6

Broccoli rabe is a popular Italian bitter green and it goes nicely with starchy white beans and potatoes. This delicious combination should be served in large, shallow soup bowls with hard-crusted Italian bread for sopping up every luscious drop of juice. Pair this dish with a bowl of steaming, fresh corn polenta and a plate of roasted peppers for an Italian vegetarian feast. I highly recommend playing Frank Sinatra's duets on the stereo while you eat this marvelous dinner.

3 medium potatoes, peeled and cut into ½-inch slices
3 tablespoons extra-virgin olive oil
5 large cloves garlic, finely chopped
2 teaspoons crushed red pepper
2 large bunches broccoli rabe, bottom 3 inches of tough stems discarded
¼ cup water
    Salt and pepper
2 cups cooked great northern or other white beans (with cooking liquid)

Cook the potatoes in lightly salted, boiling water for about 5 minutes or until fork-tender. Drain and set aside. Heat oil in a large pot over medium heat. Add garlic and crushed red pepper. Cook for 2 minutes, stirring occasionally. Add the broccoli rabe and water. Sprinkle lightly with salt and pepper. Cover and cook for about 20 minutes, stirring occasionally until the broccoli rabe is just tender. Add the cooked potatoes and the beans with their cooking liquid. Stir to combine. Continue cooking, uncovered, for 10 minutes, stirring occasionally, until heated through. Taste for seasonings.

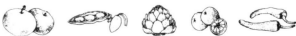

Nitin Pakoras

SERVES 4

As I was shopping in a farmer's market in Hartford, Connecticut, I commented to a fellow shopper on how huge and beautiful the bunches of cilantro were that day. I was intrigued to see that he was buying three big bunches. I had to ask him what they were for. He was making pakoras—traditional East Indian fritters—and wrote down this recipe for me, which bears his name.

- 1 cup flour
- 1 teaspoon baking powder
- 2 eggs or egg substitute, lightly beaten
- ½ cup soy milk
- 1 teaspoon plus ¼ cup peanut oil
- 1 cup finely chopped fresh cilantro
- 1 teaspoon chili powder
- 1 teaspoon cumin powder
- 1 teaspoon cumin seeds
- ½ teaspoon salt
- ½ teaspoon pepper

In a bowl, combine the flour and baking powder. Whisk together to mix. In a separate bowl, whisk together the eggs, soy milk, and 1 teaspoon of the peanut oil until well blended. Pour this into the dry ingredients all at once. Stir to combine. Stir in the cilantro, chili powder, cumin powder, cumin seeds, salt, and pepper until well blended.

Line a cookie sheet with a double thickness of paper towels. Set aside. Heat ¼ cup peanut oil in a large skillet over medium-high heat. Drop heaping tablespoons of the batter into the oil. Do not crowd the skillet or the pakoras will be greasy. Cook the pakoras for 2 to 3 minutes until golden brown. Carefully turn them, using a plastic spatula. Cook the other side for 2 to 3 minutes until golden brown. Transfer the pakoras to the paper towel-lined cookie sheet. Continue frying the remaining batter.

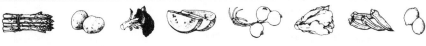

Spinach Empanadas Gallega

SERVES 6

Empanadas gallega are savory turnovers big enough for a family, and spinach is one of the many fillings you can use to create a lovely dinner pie. Serve this with Mexican Vegetables and Pinto Beans over Yellow Rice (page 238) for a great dinner.

- 1 **double unbaked crust for 9-inch pie (homemade or found in the refrigerated section of supermarkets)**
- 3 **tablespoons olive oil**
- 2 **medium sweet onions, finely chopped**
- 2 **10-ounce bags spinach, washed and finely chopped**
   Salt and pepper
- ½ **cup shredded Monterey Jack cheese**

Place one pie crust in a 9-inch glass pie plate. Set aside while you prepare the filling. Preheat the oven to 400 degrees. Heat the olive oil in a large deep skillet over medium-low heat. Add the onions. Cook for 5 minutes, stirring occasionally. Add the spinach (with the water clinging to the leaves). Sprinkle with salt and pepper to taste. Cover and cook for about 15 minutes, stirring occasionally, until the spinach is tender. Remove from the heat. Taste for seasonings. Drain the spinach in a colander set into a bowl.

Sprinkle one half of the Monterey Jack cheese evenly over the pie crust. Using a slotted spoon, transfer the cooked spinach and onions to the pie crust. Arrange the spinach evenly. Scatter the remaining Monterey Jack cheese evenly over the spinach. Place the top pie crust over the pie. Seal the edges all around by gently pressing the top and bottom crusts together using the tines of a fork. Cut four small slits into the top crust, using a sharp knife. Place the pie on a cookie sheet to catch any drippings. Bake for about 40 minutes or until the pie crust is light brown. Serve immediately or chilled.

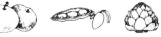

Asparagus Mini Omelettes

SERVES 8 (ABOUT 17 MINI OMELETTES)

These light little omelettes are delicious and so versatile. You can serve them with a tossed salad for lunch or brunch, and they make a lovely dinner when served with Garlic Mashed Potatoes (page 105) and Orange-Maple Carrots (page 92). In our house, we love to keep a plateful in the refrigerator—they make a terrific snack. Try them with a squeeze of fresh lemon juice on top.

  2 pounds thin asparagus, tough bottoms removed, cut into ¼-inch pieces
¼ cup olive oil
  1 medium onion, minced
  2 teaspoons water
  2 teaspoons finely grated lemon zest
10 eggs or equivalent egg substitute
  3 tablespoons minced fresh Italian flat-leaf parsley
    Salt and pepper

Cook the asparagus in lightly salted boiling water for about 5 minutes, or until tender. Drain and set aside. Heat 1 tablespoon of the olive oil in a skillet over medium heat. Add the onion. Cover and cook for 5 minutes, stirring occasionally, until softened. Add the water and lemon zest. Cover and continue cooking for 2 minutes, stirring occasionally. Remove from the heat.

Break the eggs into a medium bowl. Beat lightly with a whisk. Stir in the parsley and the sautéed onion. Add the cooked asparagus, and salt and pepper to taste. Stir well to mix.

Heat 2 teaspoons of the oil in a large, nonstick skillet over medium-high heat. Stir the omelette mixture. Using a ¼ cup measure, drop ¼ cupfuls of the omelette mixture into the heated oil, fitting as many as you can without crowding. Cook for 2 to 3 minutes or until set and golden brown, then turn each omelette over, using 2 plastic spatulas. Cook the other side for 2 to 3 minutes until golden brown. Transfer to a platter. Heat another 2 teaspoons of the oil and cook another batch. Repeat this process until all of the omelette batter is used. Serve hot or chilled.

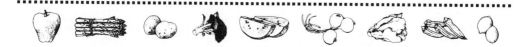

Potato, "Sausage," and Mushroom Pancakes

MAKES ABOUT 24 PANCAKES

Potatoes, meatless sausages, and mushrooms are three of my favorite foods, so it was only a matter of time before they made it into the same pan. My friends and family eat as many of these as I can make. If you can manage any leftovers, they are wonderful cold for the next day's breakfast or lunch.

    1 tablespoon extra-virgin olive oil
    ¼ pound shiitake mushrooms, stems discarded, caps thinly sliced
    5½ ounces meatless sausage, cut into ¼-inch slices
    2 teaspoons fennel seeds
    6 large potatoes
    1 medium sweet onion, finely chopped
    3 tablespoons finely chopped fresh Italian flat-leaf parsley
    6 eggs or equivalent egg substitute, lightly beaten
      Salt and pepper
    ¼ cup or more peanut oil

Heat the olive oil in a large skillet over medium heat. Add the mushrooms, meatless sausage, and fennel seeds. Cook for 10 minutes, stirring occasionally, until the mushrooms are just tender. Turn them into a mixing bowl. Peel the potatoes and drop them into a bowl of lightly salted water as you work—this will prevent them from darkening.

Line a cookie sheet with a double layer of paper towels and set it near the stove to drain the pancakes after you fry them. Grate the potatoes into a colander set in a bowl, using the large holes of a hand grater (the food processor makes them too dry). Press out as much liquid from the potatoes as you can, by pressing your hands on the potatoes against the colander. Turn the drained, grated potatoes into the mixing bowl with the sausages and mushrooms. Add the onion, parsley, eggs, and salt and pepper to taste. Stir to mix well.

Heat 2 tablespoons of the peanut oil in a large nonstick skillet over medium-high heat. Drop the pancake batter by heaping tablespoonfuls into the hot oil,

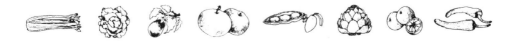

fitting as many pancakes as you can, but not crowding or the pancakes will be greasy. Fry the pancakes for about 5 minutes without turning, until they are set and golden brown. Turn and cook the other side for about 5 minutes until golden brown. Transfer the cooked pancakes onto the lined cookie sheet. Continue frying the pancakes in batches, heating additional oil as needed.

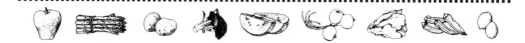

Corn-Crusted Parsnip, Sweet and White Potato Cakes

SERVES 6 (12 CAKES)

The snappy flavor of Tequila-Lime Sauce (page 122) is just perfect with these delicious little root vegetable cakes. Enjoy them served hot from the oven for dinner with a Southwestern Black Bean Salad with Chipotle-Lime Dressing (page 42) or serve them at room temperature as part of an appetizer buffet. I can assure you that if you leave a plate of these wonderful cakes on your counter, they will definitely disappear!

   3 cups Mashed Parsnips, Sweet and White Potatoes (page104)
   3 eggs or equivalent egg substitute
   1 cup cornmeal
   1 cup plain dry bread crumbs
   2 teaspoons chili powder
   ½ teaspoon dried oregano
   ¼ teaspoon ground red pepper (cayenne)
       Salt and pepper
   2 tablespoons peanut oil
       Tequila-Lime Sauce (page 122)

Have a nonstick cookie sheet ready. Fill a ¼-cup measure with the mashed parsnip mixture leveling it off with your finger. Tap the filled measuring cup onto the palm of your hand to release the contents. Gently flatten and shape this into a cake approximately 2½ inches round × ¾ inches thick. Set this on the cookie sheet and repeat the process until all 12 cakes are formed. Cover the cookie sheet with plastic wrap and refrigerate.

Beat the eggs or egg substitute in a pie dish, using a fork. In a separate pie dish, combine the cornmeal with the bread crumbs, chili powder, oregano, and ground red pepper. Sprinkle with salt and pepper to taste. Whisk together to combine. Preheat the oven to 350 degrees. Carefully dip each cake first into the beaten eggs, gently shaking off excess, then into the cornmeal mixture, carefully turning to coat both sides of each cake. As you bread each cake return it to the

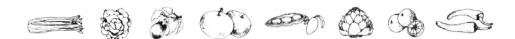

cookie sheet. When all 12 cakes are breaded, spray another cookie sheet with nonstick cooking spray and set aside.

Heat a large nonstick skillet over medium-high heat. Brush the skillet with a little peanut oil. Arrange as many cakes as you can in the skillet in a single layer, without crowding. Cook for about 4 minutes until lightly browned. Carefully turn the cakes over to brown the other side, using two plastic spatulas. Cook the other side for about 4 minutes until lightly browned. Transfer the cakes to the prepared cookie sheet. Repeat the process until all 12 cakes are browned. Bake the browned cakes for 25 minutes until heated through. Serve the cakes with Tequila-Lime Sauce.

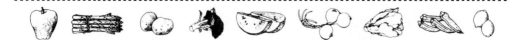

Garden Paella

SERVES 8

The marvelous aroma of saffron will fill your kitchen when you make this bountiful, traditional Spanish casserole. All you will need to serve with this glorious dish is a simple, tossed salad, some good bread, and perhaps a good Spanish wine.

⅓ cup extra-virgin olive oil

2 medium onions, chopped

3¼ cups pearl rice (Valencia) or arborio rice (both can be found in the rice or gourmet section of most supermarkets)

2 teaspoons dried thyme

2 teaspoons fennel seeds

2 bay leaves

¼ teaspoon ground red pepper (cayenne)

2 teaspoons Old Bay seasoning

1 28-ounce can Italian whole peeled tomatoes, with juice, squeezed with your hands

½ teaspoon saffron threads

½ cup dry white wine

5½ cups water

   Salt and pepper

1 medium zucchini, cut into ½-inch slices

2 medium carrots, peeled and cut into ¼-inch slices

2 ribs celery with leaves, cut into ¼-inch slices

½ cup chopped fresh Italian flat-leaf parsley

3 medium white potatoes, peeled and cut into 1-inch pieces

¼ pound string beans, cut into 1-inch pieces (about 1½ cups)

1 tablespoon capers, rinsed and squeezed dry in paper towels

1 large tomato, chopped

1 cup frozen lima beans

½ cup Spanish green olives, drained

1 cup frozen tiny green peas

1 jalapeño pepper, chopped (wash your hands immediately after handling hot peppers)

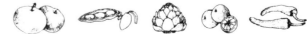

1 **cup fresh corn kernels, cut from 2 ears, *or* frozen kernels**
1 **12-ounce package meatless sausage, cut into 1-inch pieces (found in
   health food stores)**

Heat the olive oil in a large heavy pot over medium heat. Add the onions. Cover and cook for 5 minutes, stirring occasionally. Add the rice. Stir to coat. Cook for 5 minutes, stirring frequently. Lower the heat if it begins to stick. Add the thyme, fennel seeds, bay leaves, ground red pepper, and the Old Bay seasoning. Add the canned tomatoes, saffron, wine, and water. Sprinkle with salt and pepper to taste. Stir well to mix. Raise the heat to medium-high. Stir in the zucchini, carrots, celery, parsley, potatoes, string beans, capers, and the fresh tomato. Stir well to mix. Cover the pot and bring this mixture to a boil, stirring frequently so that it doesn't stick. After it reaches a boil, lower the heat to medium and continue cooking at a low-medium boil, covered, for 25 minutes, stirring frequently, until the rice and carrots are crisp-tender.

Preheat the oven to 425 degrees. Stir in the lima beans, olives, green peas, jalapeño, corn, and sausage. Stir well to combine. Spray a 4-quart casserole dish with cooking oil spray. Carefully turn the rice mixture into the prepared casserole dish. Cover tightly with foil. Bake for 1 to 1¼ hours until the rice is tender and the vegetables are tender-soft. Taste for seasonings.

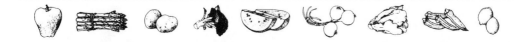

Asparagus and Tofu Pancakes

SERVES 4

These light and delicious pancakes sing of Spring's bounty. Serve them for lunch, brunch, or dinner, hot off the skillet or chilled, as is, or with lemon wedges, Marinara Sauce (page 178), applesauce, or with Portobello and Cremini Mushroom and Herb Gravy (page 123). I like them for dinner served with Garlic Mashed Potatoes (page 105) and Sweet Cinnamon Carrots (page 93).

    2 pounds asparagus, tough bottoms removed, cut into ½-inch pieces
    3 cups flour
 1½ teaspoons salt
    ⅛ teaspoon pepper
    ½ teaspoon dried dillweed
    1 tablespoon baking powder
    2 cups soy milk (found in most supermarkets and all health food stores)
    ½ pound soft tofu, drained
    ½ cup finely chopped fresh Italian flat-leaf parsley
    1 teaspoon finely grated lemon zest
    4 tablespoons olive oil

Cook the asparagus in lightly salted boiling water for about 5 minutes, or until tender-crisp. Drain. In a separate bowl, measure the flour, salt, pepper, dillweed, and baking powder. Whisk together until well mixed. Measure the soy milk and the tofu into a blender. Cover and blend on high speed for 30 seconds until well blended. Pour this mixture, all at once, over the dry ingredients. Stir lightly to combine. Stir in the asparagus, parsley, and lemon zest, mixing lightly but thoroughly.

Line a cookie sheet with a double layer of paper towels and set it by the stove. Heat 2 tablespoons of the olive oil in a large, nonstick skillet over medium heat. Drop 1 tablespoon of batter for each pancake onto the heated oil. Do not crowd or they will be greasy. Cook for 3 to 5 minutes until golden brown. Carefully turn each pancake using a plastic spatula and flatten slightly. Cook for 3 to 5 minutes until golden brown. Transfer to the paper towel-lined cookie sheet. Heat the remaining 2 tablespoons of olive oil and repeat the process until all the batter is used. Serve immediately.

Kasha with Cabbage and Portobello Mushrooms

SERVES 4

Kasha (coarsely ground buckwheat) is very traditional and popular in Russia, but with its rich nutty flavor and impressive protein and fiber content, it's becoming popular here, too—especially in my house.

2½ cups water
1 medium onion, finely chopped
3 medium carrots, peeled, cut into ¼-inch slices
1 rib celery, finely chopped
3 potatoes, peeled, cut into ½-inch cubes
 Salt and pepper
1 tablespoon olive oil
1 tablespoon soybean margarine (found in health food stores) or canola oil
½ large head green cabbage, cored and thinly sliced
3 large portobello mushroom caps (about ½ pound), cut into ⅓-inch slices
1 13-ounce box kasha (about 2¼ cups)

Place the water, onion, carrots, celery, and potatoes in a small pot. Cover and bring to a boil over high heat (this should take about 7 minutes). Lower the heat to medium. Cook, covered, at a medium boil for 10 to 12 minutes, stirring occasionally, until the potatoes are tender-crisp. Stir in salt and pepper to taste. Remove from heat and set aside. Meanwhile, heat the oil and the margarine in a 6-quart pot over medium heat. Add the cabbage and mushrooms. Sprinkle with salt and pepper. Cover and cook, stirring occasionally, for about 35 minutes until the cabbage is just tender.

Stir in the kasha. Carefully add the pot of cooked vegetables and water to the kasha. Stir well to mix. Lower the heat to low-medium. Cover and cook for about 20 minutes, stirring frequently, until the kasha is tender. Taste for seasonings.

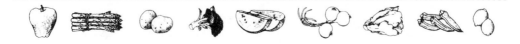

Sweet Potatoes and Kidney Beans over "Sausage" and Polenta

SERVES 6

My mom sometimes prepares this old Italian favorite for the annual summer gathering of her childhood friends, "the beach girls," and although it might not be picnic food as we know it, the flavors are wonderful. LightLife brand makes good Italian meatless links to use in this recipe.

     5 tablespoons extra-virgin olive oil
     5 large cloves garlic, minced
     5 medium sweet potatoes, peeled, cut into quarters lengthwise, then into
        ¾-inch slices
     ½ cup coarsely chopped fresh Italian flat-leaf parsley
    10 fresh basil leaves
        Salt and pepper
     2 cups cooked kidney beans, well drained
     1 10 to 12-ounce package meatless Italian sausage (found in health food
        stores), cut into ¼-inch pieces
     9 cups water
     1 medium sweet onion, finely chopped
     2 cups cornmeal

Heat 4 tablespoons of the olive oil in a large, deep skillet over low-medium heat. Add the garlic, sweet potatoes, parsley, and basil. Sprinkle with salt and pepper to taste. Cover and cook for about 35 minutes, stirring occasionally, until the potatoes are tender. Stir in the cooked beans. Taste for seasonings. Cover and keep warm. While the sweet potatoes are cooking, heat the remaining 1 tablespoon of olive oil in a medium skillet over medium-high heat. Add the sausages. Cook the sausages for 5 to 7 minutes, stirring frequently to mix, until the sausages are golden brown. Set aside while you make the polenta.

Bring the water to a boil in a 5-quart covered pot over high heat. Stir in a little salt and the onion. Cover and cook for 2 minutes. Put on oven mitts to protect your hands and arms from the hot steam. Using a long whisk, whisk the water in

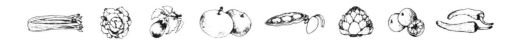

a circular motion to keep it moving. Gradually pour in the cornmeal with one hand while continually whisking with the other, stopping to whisk out the lumps if the cornmeal clumps up. Continue whisking the cornmeal until it returns to a boil, then lower the heat to medium. Cook for 2 to 3 minutes, whisking constantly, until it thickens to your liking. Whisk in salt and pepper to taste. Turn the polenta onto a large, deep serving platter. Spoon the cooked sweet potatoes and kidney beans with the juices evenly over the polenta, leaving a 1-inch border around the polenta. Scatter the browned sausages over the top. Serve immediately or at room temperature.

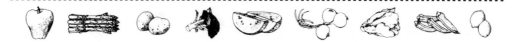

Stewed White Beans with Spinach, Onions, and Garlic Toasts

SERVES 8

Serve this richly flavored Italian stew in large rimmed bowls, then break Little Garlic Toasts (page 81) into chunks and drop them into each bowl. Next, use a potato peeler to make curls of Romano cheese to place on top of each steaming bowlful of soup. Let the crunchy little toasts absorb the delicious broth and the Romano cheese melt into the soup ever so slightly. Then sprinkle a little fresh black pepper on top, and enjoy one of the greatest treats your nose and mouth can have. If they could, they'd send you a thank you note.

  1 pound white kidney beans, picked over for stones
2½ quarts (10 cups) water
  1 bay leaf
    Salt and pepper
 ¼ cup extra-virgin olive oil
  1 large sweet onion, coarsely chopped
  1 large red (Bermuda) onion, coarsely chopped
 ½ teaspoon crushed red pepper
  1 pound fresh spinach, well washed and coarsely chopped
  1 recipe Little Garlic Toasts (page 81)
    Romano cheese curls

Put the beans and water into a large heavy pot. Add the bay leaf, cover the pot, and place over high heat. When it comes to a rapid boil, lower the heat to low-medium. Cook, covered, at a low-medium boil for 1½ hours, stirring occasionally. Stir in a little salt and pepper to taste. Cover and continue cooking at a medium boil, stirring occasionally, for another 30 minutes or until the beans are tender-soft.

Meanwhile, heat the olive oil in a large skillet over low-medium heat. Add the onions and crushed red pepper. Sprinkle lightly with salt and pepper and stir to mix. Cover and cook for 10 minutes, stirring occasionally, until the onions are

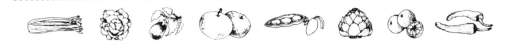

softened and have released their liquids. Add the spinach. Sprinkle lightly with salt and pepper. Cover and cook for 10 to 12 minutes, stirring occasionally, until the spinach is wilted. Remove from the heat and set aside until the beans are fully cooked. When the beans are tender-soft, remove the bay leaf and stir the cooked spinach and onions into the beans, using a rubber spatula to scrape all of the spinach and juices into the pot. Stir well to combine and to heat through. Taste for seasonings. To serve, pass the Little Garlic Toasts, Romano cheese curls, and black pepper.

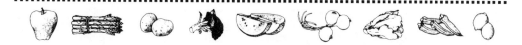

Cauliflower with Angel Hair Pasta in a Light Broth with Parmesan Cheese

SERVES 8

One of the many wonderful benefits of my first cookbook was the opportunity to meet fellow food-lovers. During a book signing in Florida, I met Bernadette Misuraca, a generous cook who told me about this delicately flavored, old Italian combination of angel hair pasta cooked in water in which you first cook cauliflower. The result is just lovely. I serve it in large bowls with a side dish of Roasted Bell Peppers with Capers, Olives, and Oregano (page 78) and a simple tossed salad. Pass around plenty of fresh pepper, grated Parmesan cheese, and good bread for dunking. Great ideas come from kind people everywhere!

    1 large head of cauliflower (about 2½ pounds), with greens attached
    3 quarts plus 2 cups water
    1 bay leaf
       Salt and pepper
    1 pound angel hair pasta (capellini), broken into little pieces
    ¼ cup extra-virgin olive oil
    8 large cloves garlic, coarsely chopped
    1 cup finely chopped fresh Italian flat-leaf parsley
       Grated Parmesan cheese, optional

Place the cauliflower, water, and the bay leaf in an 8-quart pot. Sprinkle with salt and pepper to taste. Cover and bring to a boil over high heat; lower the heat to medium. Cook, covered, at a medium boil until fork-tender, about 30 minutes. Turn the cauliflower over occasionally, using two large slotted spoons, to cook evenly. When cooked, using the two slotted spoons carefully lift the cauliflower out of the cooking liquid and into a bowl. Set aside. Remove the bay leaf. Raise the heat under the cauliflower cooking liquid to high. When the liquid comes to a full boil, stir in the broken angel hair pasta. Cook until tender. Cover and lower the heat to simmer to keep warm while you sauté the cauliflower.

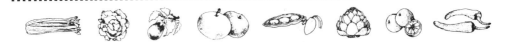

When the cauliflower is cool enough to handle, remove and discard the green leaves and the core, using your hands. Break the cauliflower into little pieces. It should come apart quite easily. Heat the olive oil in a medium-size skillet over low-medium heat. Add the cauliflower, garlic, and parsley. Cover and cook for 15 minutes, stirring occasionally.

Pour this mixture into the pasta and broth, scraping the pan with a spoon to remove all of the juices. Stir well to mix. Taste for seasonings. To serve, ladle into serving bowls, top each bowl with freshly ground black pepper, and pass the grated Parmesan cheese.

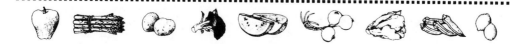

Potatoes and Eggs

SERVES 4

I always thought of potatoes and eggs as an Italian dish. I knew it as the frittata that we often ate on Friday nights during Lent, particularly at my mother-in-law's house. Then I learned from my friend Alberto, from Madrid, that this is a traditional Spanish dish, too—but they call it a tortilla. By any name, it is one of my favorite dishes. It's the perfect dinner when you don't think you have any-thing in the house to cook. And leftovers are wonderful for breakfast or for the next day's lunch in a sandwich with a little ketchup. Serve it for dinner with left-over Roasted Bell Peppers with Capers, Olives, and Oregano (page 78), Fresh Tomato Salad (page 54), or another salad topped with a handful of cooked chick-peas and bread for a lovely meal.

2 tablespoons extra-virgin olive oil
1 medium onion, finely chopped
3 medium potatoes, peeled and thinly sliced
   Salt and pepper
8 beaten eggs or equivalent egg substitute

Heat the oil in a medium nonstick skillet over medium heat. Add the onions, then arrange the potatoes over the onions. Sprinkle with salt and pepper. Cover and cook without disturbing for 10 minutes, until tender. Test the potatoes for doneness, using a fork. If they are tender, proceed; if not cover and continue cooking for another 3 to 4 minutes. Stir the potatoes and onions to mix. Pour the beaten eggs evenly over the potatoes and onions. Sprinkle with salt and pepper. Cover and cook for about 12 minutes, until the eggs are just set.

Carefully place a large plate (the size of the skillet) over the top of the skillet. Wear a pair of oven mitts while you turn the potatoes and eggs onto the plate by flipping the skillet over while holding the plate firmly. Slide the "pancake" back into the skillet, the uncooked side down. Continue cooking, uncovered, for 4 to 6 minutes until the eggs are cooked. Test for doneness by gently lifting the edges using a plastic spatula. Carefully slide the potato and egg "pancake" from the skillet onto a large serving plate. Cut into 4 wedges.

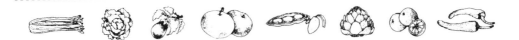

Grandma McHugh's Baked Beans with Meatless Hot Dogs

SERVES 8

My good friend Claudia's family has lived in New England for generations. She was generous enough to share several of her Old New England baked bean recipes with me, and this is her grandmother's recipe—with a few additions! Tofu dogs add a luscious, smoky flavor to this delicious, molasses-flavored dish.

- 2 quarts water
- 12 ounces (1½ cups) navy pea beans, picked over for stones
- 1 bay leaf
- ½ cup blackstrap molasses
- 1 medium onion, finely chopped
- ¼ cup firmly packed brown sugar
- 3 ounces meatless bacon (found in health food stores), cut into 1-inch pieces
- ¼ cup ketchup
- ¼ cup pure maple syrup
- 3 tablespoons Dijon mustard
- Salt and pepper
- 12 ounces meatless hot dogs (found in health food stores and most supermarkets)

Place the water, beans, and bay leaf in a large pot over high heat. Cover and bring to a boil. When it comes to a full boil, reduce the heat to medium. Continue cooking, covered, at a medium boil for 1¼ hours, stirring occasionally.

Preheat the oven to 400 degrees. Add the molasses, onion, brown sugar, meatless bacon, ketchup, maple syrup, and mustard to the beans. Stir well to mix. Stir in salt and pepper to taste. Spray a 3-quart glass casserole dish with nonstick cooking spray. Turn the bean mixture into the prepared casserole dish, using a rubber spatula to scrape all of the contents from the pot. Cover tightly with foil. Bake for 1¾ hours. Remove the foil. Stir to mix. Continue baking, uncovered, for about 1 hour, stirring occasionally, until the beans are tender. Add the meatless hot dogs, pushing them into the casserole using a spoon, until they are covered by the beans. Continue baking, uncovered, for about 5 minutes until the hot dogs are heated through. Remove the bay leaf.

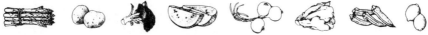

6
Desserts

- Plantain-Date Bread
- Chocolate Crepes with Bananas and a Strawberry Purée
- Dairy-Free Gingerbread
- Parsnip Cake
- Dairy-Free Chocolate-Zucchini Cake
- Dairy-Free Chocolate-Almond Cake
- Pumpkin-Ricotta Cheese Pie
- Dairy-Free Pumpkin Pie
- Maple-Tofu Pie
- Italian Chocolate Spice Cookies
- Muzzet
- Butterballs
- All-American Fresh Fruit Cobbler
- Pumpkin Cookies with Currants and Chocolate Chips
- Flan
- Stewed Chestnuts
- Pumpkin Bread Pudding
- Apricot-Peach Purée
- Peaches in Merlot
- Lemon Frosting
- Chocolate Glaze

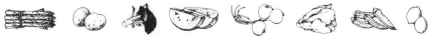

Plantain-Date Bread

MAKES ONE 12-CUP BUNDT

Plantains are wonderfully versatile Latin American bananas that must be cooked before eating. They have become so popular that most supermarkets carry them year-round. Buy yellow (ripe) plantains for this wonderful bread and serve it for breakfast or dessert, or use it to make sandwiches with fat-free or non-dairy cream cheese from the health food store.

- 1 cup sugar
- ½ cup Spectrum spread, a nonhydrogenated vegetable shortening (found in health food stores)
- 2 eggs or egg substitute, lightly beaten
- 3 ripe plantains, mashed (about 2 cups)
- ½ cup chopped walnuts
- ½ cup chopped dates
- 2 cups flour
- 1 teaspoon baking soda

Preheat the oven to 350 degrees. Cream the sugar and the Spectrum spread in a bowl, beating with a wooden spoon. Add the eggs and beat well to combine. Stir in the mashed plantains, walnuts, and dates. In a separate bowl, whisk together the flour and the baking soda. Add this to the creamed mixture. Stir well to combine. Spray a 12-cup Bundt pan with nonstick cooking spray. Turn the batter into the prepared pan, using a rubber spatula to scrape the bowl. Bake for about 1 hour and 15 minutes or until a cake tester inserted into the center comes out fairly clean and the bread pulls away from the sides of the pan. Serve warm or at room temperature.

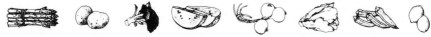

Chocolate Crepes with Bananas and a Strawberry Purée

SERVES 8

This is a perfectly delicious ending to any meal, but tastes particularly good after a Mexican-inspired dinner. What a luscious way to enjoy the benefits of soy and fresh fruits!

Crepes:

 2 eggs or equivalent egg substitute
½ cup minus 1 tablespoon soy milk
½ cup minus 1 tablespoon rice milk
 2 tablespoons chocolate liqueur (Godiva is my favorite)
½ teaspoon pure vanilla extract
½ cup flour
¼ cup sugar
 2 tablespoons unsweetened cocoa
¼ teaspoon cinnamon

Strawberry Purée:

 1 pint fresh strawberries, cut in half
 1 tablespoon sugar
 2 tablespoons rice milk

Filling:

 4 bananas
½ cup chocolate syrup (store bought is fine)

Measure the eggs, soy milk, rice milk, chocolate liqueur, and vanilla into a blender. Cover and blend on high speed for 10 seconds. Measure the flour, sugar, cocoa, and cinnamon into a sifter set in a bowl. Sift to combine. Spoon the flour mixture into the blender. Cover and blend on high speed for 10 seconds, until the mixture is smooth, stopping once to scrape down the sides. Pour this mixture into a bowl and set aside while you make the strawberry purée.

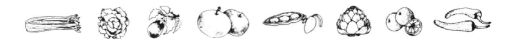

Place the strawberries, sugar, and rice milk in the clean blender cup. Cover. Pulse 15 to 20 times, stopping once or twice to mix, until the mixture is blended and chunky. Set aside while you cook the crepes.

Line two cookie sheets with wax paper and set them near the stove. Heat a 10-inch nonstick skillet over low-medium heat. Spray the skillet with cooking spray. Ladle or dip up ¼ cup of batter and pour into the skillet, tilting the pan to coat the bottom in a free-form circle. Cook for about 30 seconds. Carefully turn the crepe over to cook the other side, using a plastic spatula. Cook for 30 seconds. The crepe will be set. Transfer the crepe to the wax paper-lined cookie sheet. Repeat this process until you have used all of the batter. Arrange the crepes in a single layer on the wax paper as you cook them. You will make about 9 crepes.

Assemble the crepes: Peel the bananas. Cut each banana in half lengthwise. Cut each half into 4 spears. Set aside. Pour about ¼ cup of strawberry purée onto a dessert plate. Set a crepe on top. Arrange 4 banana spears in a double row down the center of the crepe. Fold each side over the center, covering the banana spears. Drizzle about a tablespoon of chocolate syrup in a zig-zag pattern over the crepe. Repeat with the remaining crepes until you have 8 marvelous desserts, plus 1 extra crepe for the cook!

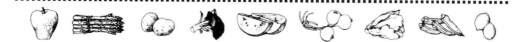

Dairy-Free Gingerbread

SERVES 8 (ONE 8-INCH PAN)

This is one of my favorite desserts, and one of the oldest I know of—I've seen recipes dating back to the early fifteenth century. I love molasses and I am especially happy to eat a calcium-rich treat with the added benefit of tofu. Although I prefer my gingerbread plain, when I was growing up, my neighbor Millie Riccitelli used to serve her gingerbread with a lemon topping, and the combination is quite popular. Try it with my Lemon Frosting (page 290).

1½ cups flour
 1 teaspoon ground ginger
¼ teaspoon salt
¼ teaspoon cinnamon
 1 teaspoon baking powder
¼ cup hot water
 3 tablespoons softened soybean margarine (found in health food stores)
 1 teaspoon baking soda
¼ cup soft tofu, drained
 1 cup blackstrap molasses

Preheat the oven to 350 degrees. Measure the flour, ginger, salt, cinnamon, and baking powder into a bowl. Whisk together to mix well. Put the hot water, margarine, baking soda, tofu, and the molasses into a blender. Cover and blend on high speed for 30 seconds until blended well. Pour this mixture all at once over the dry ingredients, using a rubber spatula to scrape the blender. Stir the ingredients together, using a wooden spoon, for about 1 minute until all of the ingredients are blended. Spray an 8-inch glass baking pan with nonstick cooking spray. Pour the batter into the prepared pan, using a rubber spatula to scrape the bowl. Smooth the top using the spatula. Bake for 40 to 45 minutes until a tester inserted into the center comes out clean. Serve warm or at room temperature.

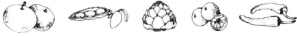

Parsnip Cake

MAKES ONE 12-CUP BUNDT CAKE

Carrot cake, zucchini cake, and now parsnip cake—what next? I can hardly wait!

- 2¼ cups flour
- 1¼ cups sugar
- 4 teaspoons baking powder
- ¼ teaspoon salt
- ½ teaspoon cinnamon
- ¼ teaspoon nutmeg
- 3 eggs or egg substitute
- ½ cup canola oil
- ⅓ cup soy milk
- 1½ cups peeled, grated parsnips (about 2 large parsnips)
- 1 tablespoon finely grated lemon zest

Preheat the oven to 350 degrees. Measure the flour, sugar, baking powder, salt, cinnamon, and nutmeg into a large bowl. Whisk together to combine. In a separate bowl, whisk together the eggs, oil, and soy milk until well blended. Pour this over the dry ingredients, all at once. Stir to mix well. Stir in the parsnips and the lemon zest until thoroughly combined. Spray a 12-cup Bundt pan with nonstick cooking spray. Pour the batter into the prepared pan, using a rubber spatula to scrape the bowl. Bake for 45 minutes or until a cake tester inserted into the center comes out clean.

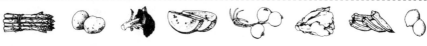

Dairy-Free Chocolate-Zucchini Cake

MAKES ONE 12-CUP BUNDT CAKE

My aunt Jerry is one of the finest, most creative bakers I know and over the years I have been one of her most enthusiastic consumers. She was way ahead of her time when she started to venture into unusual combinations (chocolate and zucchini?) in both her cooking and her baking. In this case, you'll see, smell, and taste that chocolate and zucchini were meant to be together.

2¼ cups flour
 4 teaspoons baking powder
 ¼ teaspoon salt
1⅔ cups sugar
 1 cup unsweetened cocoa
 ½ cup canola oil
 ⅔ cup soft tofu, crumbled and drained
 1 cup soy milk
 1 teaspoon pure vanilla extract
 2 medium zucchini, coarsely grated, liquid included
 1 tablespoon finely grated lemon zest
 ½ cup finely chopped prunes (oil your knife before chopping)

Preheat the oven to 350 degrees. Measure the flour, baking powder, salt, sugar, and cocoa into a bowl. Sift the ingredients into a mixing bowl. Measure the canola oil, tofu, soy milk, and vanilla extract into a blender. Cover the blender and blend on high speed for 1 minute, stopping once to scrape down the sides using a rubber spatula. Pour this over the dry ingredients all at once, using a rubber spatula to scrape the blender. Stir in the zucchini, lemon zest, and prunes, mixing well to combine.

Spray a 12-cup Bundt pan with nonstick cooking spray. Turn the batter into the prepared pan, using a rubber spatula to scrape the bowl. Bake for about 1½ hours, until the sides of the cake pull away from the pan. Serve warm or at room temperature. This cake keeps well for up to 4 days when wrapped in foil.

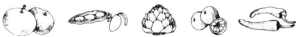

Dairy-Free Chocolate-Almond Cake

MAKES ONE 12-CUP BUNDT CAKE

This delicious cake is enriched with both tofu and soy milk, and if you ever doubted that a tofu dessert could taste luscious, you're in for a big surprise.

2¼ cups unbleached white flour
4 teaspoons baking powder
¼ teaspoon salt
1⅔ cups sugar
1 cup unsweetened cocoa
½ cup (1 stick) soybean margarine, softened to room temperature (found in health food stores)
⅔ cup soft tofu, crumbled and drained
1¼ cups soy milk
1 teaspoon pure almond extract
1 cup slivered almonds

Preheat the oven to 350 degrees. Measure the flour, baking powder, salt, sugar, and cocoa into a bowl. Sift them together into a large mixing bowl. Measure the soy margarine, tofu, soy milk, and almond extract into a blender. Cover and blend on low speed for 5 seconds. Stop to scrape down sides using a rubber spatula. Cover and blend on high speed for 1 minute, stopping once to scrape down the sides. Pour the blended ingredients over the dry ingredients all at once. Beat lightly with a wooden spoon for about 30 seconds to mix. Stir in almonds. Spray a 10-inch Bundt pan with nonstick cooking spray. Turn the batter into the prepared pan, using a rubber spatula to scrape the bowl. Spread the batter smooth. Bake for about 50 minutes until a tester inserted into the center comes out clean. Remove the pan from the oven and let set for 2 minutes before turning onto a cake dish.

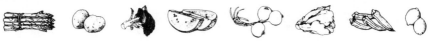

Pumpkin-Ricotta Cheese Pie

SERVES 6

*We first began making this delicious pie at **Claire's** when we had small amounts of both our pumpkin pie and our traditional Italian ricotta cheese pie fillings left over, and neither was enough to make an entire pie. Together they made one scrumptious pie that became a delectable Italian-American favorite.*

3 eggs or equivalent egg substitute
1 cup pumpkin purée, canned or fresh
½ cup ricotta cheese
½ cup sugar
1 teaspoon baking powder
1 teaspoon cinnamon
1 tablespoon flour
½ cup plus 2 tablespoons soy milk
1 teaspoon pure vanilla extract
1 9-inch unbaked pie crust (a good store-bought one is fine)

Preheat the oven to 375 degrees. Combine the eggs, pumpkin purée, ricotta cheese, sugar, baking powder, cinnamon, flour, soy milk, and vanilla in a mixing bowl. Whisk together until well blended. Place the pie crust on a cookie sheet to catch any drippings. Pour the filling into the pie crust, using a rubber spatula to scrape the bowl. Bake for about 1 hour until the center is set. Serve warm or chilled.

Dairy-Free Pumpkin Pie

SERVES 6

I used to eat pumpkin pies only around Thanksgiving. That was before I knew of the nutritional importance of beta-carotene, of which pumpkins are a rich and delicious source. Here is a luscious dessert you can proudly serve year-round.

    1 16-ounce can pumpkin (about 2 cups)
    1 cup sugar
  ¼ teaspoon salt
    1 teaspoon cinnamon
  ½ teaspoon ginger
  ⅛ teaspoon nutmeg
  ½ cup soft tofu, drained and crumbled
    2 cups soy milk (found in most supermarkets and all health food stores)
    1 10-inch prebaked pie crust (store bought or homemade)

Preheat oven to 375 degrees. Measure the pumpkin, sugar, salt, cinnamon, ginger, and nutmeg into a bowl. Whisk together until well mixed. Into a blender, measure the tofu and the soy milk. Cover and blend on high speed for 15 seconds until well blended. Pour this, all at once, into the pumpkin mixture. Whisk together for about 30 seconds until well mixed. Place the pie crust on a cookie sheet to collect any spills. Pour the pumpkin mixture into the crust, using a rubber spatula to scrape the bowl. Smooth the top with the rubber spatula. Bake for 1 hour until the center is set. Let set for 30 minutes before serving, or chill until ready to serve.

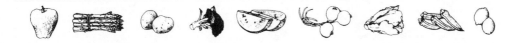

Maple-Tofu Pie

SERVES 6

Debbie Rhine, one of the many talented members of the original **Claire's** *staff from back in the late seventies, taught me a great deal about vegetarian cooking. She often made tofu pies. Unfortunately, most people back then weren't terribly interested in tofu dishes, and certainly not tofu desserts. Debbie made them anyway, because she and I enjoyed eating them. Well, of course, it turns out that tofu and soy products are extremely good for you. I always knew they were great-tasting! If you haven't tasted tofu since then, give this recipe a chance. Try topping it with Apricot-Peach Purée (page 288).*

  1 pound soft tofu, drained and crumbled
  1 cup soy milk
  ¼ cup pure maple syrup
  1 lime, squeezed, about 1½ tablespoons juice
  1 8-inch graham cracker pie crust or other prebaked pie crust

Preheat the oven to 375 degrees. Place the tofu, soy milk, maple syrup, and lime juice in a blender. Cover. Blend on high speed for 5 seconds, then pulse about 5 times for one second each until the filling is smooth.

Pour into the pie crust, using a rubber spatula to scrape the sides of the blender. Smooth the filling, using a rubber spatula. Bake the pie for 1 hour and 5 minutes. Remove from oven. Let set for 30 minutes, then chill until ready to serve.

Italian Chocolate Spice Cookies

MAKES ABOUT 6 DOZEN COOKIES

I'm thrilled whenever I receive an invitation to a party at my aunt Marge's house. It's always a pleasure to share a happy occasion with the family, but I shamefully admit that when I open the invitation, my immediate thoughts are of the delicious, rich, Italian chocolate cookies Aunt Marge has become famous for.

    4 cups flour
    2 cups sugar
    1 cup unsweetened cocoa
    2 teaspoons baking powder
1½ teaspoons cinnamon
1½ teaspoons ground cloves
    1 egg or equivalent egg substitute
    1 large orange, squeezed, about 1 cup juice
    ½ cup soybean oil
1¼ cups soy milk
       Chocolate Glaze (page 290), optional

Preheat the oven to 350 degrees. Measure the flour, sugar, cocoa, baking powder, cinnamon, and cloves into a bowl. Stir to mix. Sift the dry ingredients into another bowl. In a separate bowl, whisk together the egg, orange juice, oil, and milk until well blended. Pour the liquid ingredients over the dry, all at once. Stir well to mix thoroughly. The batter will be quite thick. Spray 2 cookie sheets with nonstick cooking spray or line with parchment paper. Drop the batter by heaping teaspoonfuls in rows (about 3 rows by 4 rows), leaving about 1 inch between the cookies. Bake for about 13 minutes, until a cake tester inserted into the center of a cookie comes out clean. Remove from the oven. Set aside until cooled to room temperature. Drizzle with Chocolate Glaze, if desired. Store in a covered container for up to one week.

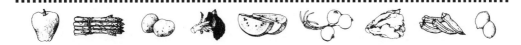

Muzzet

MAKES ABOUT 7 DOZEN COOKIES

My aunt Connie makes the most delicious and tender muzzet, flavorful Italian cookies that you just can't stop eating. They are perfect for dunking into a cup of espresso or a glass of cold soy milk.

2 cups vegetable shortening
2 cups sugar
6 eggs or egg substitute, plus 1 for brushing tops of loaves
2 tablespoons pure vanilla extract
2 tablespoons finely grated orange zest
1 tablespoon finely grated lemon zest
6 cups flour
2 tablespoons baking powder
½ pound sliced almonds

Preheat the oven to 325 degrees. Cream the shortening and sugar together in a large bowl, using a wooden spoon to beat the combination smooth. One at a time, beat in 6 eggs, beating smooth after each addition. Beat in the vanilla and orange and lemon zest. Into a separate bowl, measure the flour and baking powder. Whisk to combine. Add to the creamed mixture. Stir together to mix thoroughly. Spray 2 cookie sheets with nonstick cooking spray or line the cookie sheets with parchment paper. Form the dough into 4 small loaves, 8 × 5 × 1-inch each. Arrange 2 small loaves on each prepared cookie sheet, leaving space in between each. Lightly beat the remaining egg in a small bowl. Lightly brush the tops of each loaf with the beaten egg, trying not to allow the egg to drip onto the cookie sheet or the loaves will stick. Scatter the sliced almonds evenly over the loaves. Bake for about 45 minutes until the loaves are golden brown and a cake tester inserted into the center comes out clean. Set aside to cool before cutting each loaf in half lengthwise, then into ¾- to 1-inch slices. Store in a covered tin or jar for up to one week.

Butterballs

MAKES ABOUT 33 COOKIES

In my family, we always associated certain desserts with certain aunts. Aunt Connie made the Muzzet (page 280), Aunt Marge made the Italian Chocolate Spice Cookies (page 279), and Aunt Louise made the Butterballs for our family celebrations. In fact, to this day, I can't imagine a bridal or baby shower or a christening without these delicate, melt-in-your-mouth cookies. You really need to splurge and use real butter in this recipe—they just won't taste the same without it.

> 1 cup (2 sticks) butter, softened to room temperature
> 2 cups confectioners' sugar
> 1 teaspoon pure vanilla extract
> 1¾ cups flour
> ¼ cup finely chopped walnuts

Preheat the oven to 350 degrees. Beat the butter and 1 cup of the confectioners' sugar together until smooth, using a wooden spoon. Beat in the vanilla. Add the flour. Stir well to mix thoroughly. Stir in the walnuts, mixing well to combine. Take a heaping teaspoonful of the cookie batter into your hand. Roll it into a bite-size ball. Place on an ungreased cookie sheet. Roll all of the cookie batter into balls. Arrange the butterballs on the cookie sheet, leaving a little space in between each. Bake for 15 to 18 minutes until golden brown. Remove from the oven. Let cool for 30 minutes. Place the remaining cup of confectioners' sugar in a bowl. Carefully but thoroughly roll the butterballs, one at a time, in the sugar, coating completely. Gently shake off any excess. Arrange the butterballs on a platter or in a covered tin. If they are covered tightly, they will keep for up to two weeks.

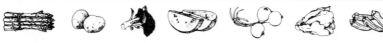

All-American Fresh Fruit Cobbler

SERVES 10

Red strawberries, crisp white-fleshed apples, and juicy blueberries make this delicious dessert a year-round all-American favorite.

    12 medium baking apples, such as Rome Beauty or Cortland
     1 pint blueberries, picked over
     1 quart strawberries, hulled
    ½ cup firmly packed brown sugar
    ¼ cup white sugar
     1 tablespoon cinnamon
    ½ lemon, squeezed, about 2 tablespoons juice
    ¼ cup water

Topping:

    1½ cups flour
    ½ cup rolled oats
    ¼ cup wheat germ
     2 teaspoons baking powder
     1 tablespoon grated lemon zest
     2 eggs or egg substitute, lightly beaten
    ½ cup white sugar
    ¼ cup soybean margarine (½ stick), melted (found in health food stores)
     1 cup soy milk

Preheat the oven to 350 degrees. Core and peel the apples, then cut them in half and cut each half into ¼-inch slices. Place the apples in a large bowl. Add the blueberries and strawberries. Toss gently to mix, using two wooden spoons. Add the brown sugar, white sugar, cinnamon, lemon juice, and water. Toss gently but thoroughly to mix. Spray a 3-quart glass baking dish with nonstick cooking spray. Turn the fruit into the prepared baking dish, using a rubber spatula to scrape the bowl.

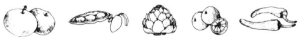

Prepare the topping: Measure the flour, oats, wheat germ, baking powder, and lemon zest into a bowl. Whisk together to mix. Into a separate bowl, measure the eggs, sugar, margarine, and soy milk. Whisk together until well blended. Pour the liquid ingredients over the dry ingredients, all at once. Stir to mix until blended. Pour the cobbler topping evenly over the fruit filling. Bake for about 1½ hours until the fruit is bubbly and the topping is golden brown.

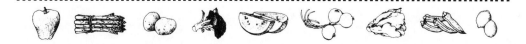

Pumpkin Cookies with Currants and Chocolate Chips

MAKES 4 DOZEN

These cookies were an instant success at my house and in my restaurant on the day Rose Albin brought in her mom's recipe for us to try.

1 cup canola oil
2 eggs or equivalent egg substitute
2 cups sugar
4 cups flour
1 16-ounce can pumpkin purée
2 teaspoons cinnamon
2 teaspoons baking soda
2 tablespoons soy milk
2 teaspoons pure vanilla extract
4 teaspoons baking powder
1 cup chocolate chips
1 cup currants

Preheat the oven to 375 degrees. Combine all of the ingredients in a mixing bowl. Mix until well combined, using a wooden spoon. Do not overbeat or your cookies will be tough. Spray 2 cookie sheets with nonstick cooking spray. Drop the dough by heaping teaspoonfuls onto the sheets in well-spaced rows, leaving about 1 inch between the cookies. Bake for 12 minutes or until just firm to the touch.

Flan

SERVES 8

The manager of my building, Juan Vega, promised me that his mother's flan recipe was better than any other and he was not exaggerating. This flan is the best! It is probably the richest, too—save it for special occasions and savor every mouthful.

1 12-ounce can evaporated milk
1 14-ounce can sweetened condensed milk
4 eggs
2 teaspoons pure vanilla extract
1 teaspoon sugar
1 8-ounce package cream cheese, cut into small cubes

Syrup:

1 cup sugar

Preheat the oven to 350 degrees. Measure the evaporated milk, condensed milk, eggs, vanilla, sugar, and cream cheese into a blender. Cover and blend on low speed for 5 seconds. Scrape down the sides with a rubber spatula. Cover and blend on high speed for 20 seconds, stopping once to scrape down the sides, until the mixture is smooth and creamy. Spray an 11-inch glass baking dish with non-stick cooking spray.

Make the syrup: Measure the sugar into a small pot. Place over low heat and bring to a low boil, stirring occasionally, until the color turns golden brown. Don't let the syrup turn dark brown or it will taste bitter. Remove the pot from the heat immediately. Quickly (it hardens fast) pour the syrup into the prepared glass baking dish, using a rubber spatula to scrape the pot. Spread the syrup evenly on the bottom of the dish. Pour the contents of the blender over the syrup, using a rubber spatula to scrape the blender. Smooth the top. Set the baking dish into a larger baking dish. Pour 3 cups of hot water into the larger baking dish to fill to about half the depth of the smaller baking dish. Bake for about 1 hour until the flan is golden brown and a knife inserted into the center comes out clean. Serve immediately or chilled. Spoon the juices over the flan as you serve it.

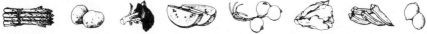

Stewed Chestnuts

SERVES 8

For as long as I've known my husband Frank, he has talked about the wonderful stewed chestnut dessert that his grandmother, who was born in southern Italy, used to make when he was a child. I can't imagine what took me so long to try to duplicate this simple dish, but Frank is certainly happy that I did finally get around to it, and so am I. You can buy whole peeled chestnuts in cans at gourmet markets and in the specialty section of some supermarkets, which is a real time- and work-saver. Chestnuts are delicious and rich in fiber, so I make stewed chest- nuts a part of every fall season at our house. We serve them in wine glasses.

    1 20-ounce (approximately) can whole chestnuts in water
    2 cups water
    ½ cup sugar
    1 bay leaf

Stir together the chestnuts with their liquid, the water, sugar, and bay leaf in a pot. Cover and bring to a boil over high heat. Lower the heat to low-medium and cook, uncovered, at a low boil for 1 hour, until the liquid is syrupy. Remove the bay leaf. Taste for sweetness, adding more sugar if necessary. Serve immediately or chilled.

Pumpkin Bread Pudding

SERVES 6

Bread pudding has recently made a strong comeback, appearing on the dessert menus of even the most sophisticated restaurants. How nice to see comfort food making it to the big time.

  1 16-ounce can pumpkin (about 2 cups)
  ½ cup firmly packed brown sugar
  1 teaspoon cinnamon
  1 teaspoon pure vanilla extract
  ¼ teaspoon nutmeg
  6 eggs or equivalent egg substitute
  4 cups soy-rice milk (found in health food stores)
  6 1-inch-thick slices French or Italian bread, each slice torn into 5 to 6 pieces
  ½ cup golden raisins

Preheat the oven to 350 degrees. Combine the pumpkin, brown sugar, cinnamon, vanilla, and nutmeg in a large bowl. Mix thoroughly using a whisk. Add the eggs and the soy-rice milk. Whisk together until well blended. Add the bread and raisins. Stir to mix. Push the bread and the raisins down into the liquid, using a wooden spoon. Let set for 30 minutes, pushing the bread and raisins down if they float to the surface. Spray a 3-quart glass baking dish with nonstick cooking spray. Turn the pumpkin bread pudding into the prepared baking dish, using a rubber spatula to scrape the bowl. Bake for about 1½ hours until set. Test for doneness by scooping out a spoonful of pudding from the center. Bake until the eggs are fully cooked and set. Serve immediately or chilled.

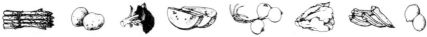

Apricot-Peach Purée

MAKES ABOUT 2½ CUPS

I just love it when something so easy to prepare can also turn a humble tofu pie, a plain cake, or even fat-free frozen yogurt into an elegant dessert. The real plus is that this purée is rich in fiber, vitamins, and beta-carotene. Dessert doesn't get much better than this.

- 4 large ripe apricots, pitted
- 4 large ripe peaches
- ½ small orange squeezed, or ¼ cup good orange juice
- 1 teaspoon pure almond extract or hazelnut liqueur (either is wonderful with the apricots and peaches)

Slice the apricots into thirds. Place the apricots in a small pot. Peel and pit the peaches. Do this right over the pot with the apricots so that the sweet juices will drip into the pot. Slice the peaches and add them to the pot. Add the orange juice. Cover the pot and cook over low heat for 15 to 20 minutes, stirring occasionally, until the apricots and peaches are tender to soft. Mash this mixture into a slightly chunky consistency, using a potato masher. Stir in the extract or liqueur. Taste for sweetness. If you prefer a sweeter purée, stir in a teaspoon or two of sugar until it reaches your preference.

Peaches in Merlot

SERVES 6 TO 8

My grandmother made this traditional Italian dessert every summer when plump, juicy, sweet peaches filled the markets. Grandma used the sweet red wine that Grandpa made each year. I don't always have homemade red wine available these days, although my brother Paul now makes it, so I use Merlot, which I generally keep in good supply for serving with dinner and for this recipe. Serve these delicious peaches alone or on top of angel food cake for a perfect ending to a wonderful Italian meal.

    8 large ripe peaches (about 3½ pounds)
    2 tablespoons sugar
    ½ cup Merlot (or homemade red wine)

Pit peaches and slice them 1-inch thick. Place in a bowl with any juices. Sprinkle with sugar. Toss gently to mix. Pour the wine over the peaches and toss gently to mix. Set aside, unrefrigerated, for 1 hour, gently tossing every 15 minutes or so to combine flavors. Serve immediately or cover and refrigerate (I use a glass jar) for up to 3 days.

Lemon Frosting

MAKES A LITTLE OVER 1 CUP, ENOUGH TO FROST AN 8 × 8-INCH CAKE

This dairy-free, lemony frosting has the consistency of a glaze and is delicious on gingerbread, lemon poppyseed cake, or any pound cake.

2½ cups confectioners' sugar
 1 teaspoon finely grated lemon zest
 1 lemon, squeezed, about 3 tablespoons juice
 2 tablespoons soy milk

Sift the sugar into a small bowl. Add the lemon zest, lemon juice, and soy milk. Beat with a wooden spoon until soft and creamy. Spoon over a cooled cake, allowing it to drizzle down the sides.

Chocolate Glaze

MAKES ABOUT 1¼ CUPS

This glaze is delicious drizzled on top of Italian Chocolate Spice Cookies (page 271), or on top of any cake or cookie for that matter.

 2 cups sifted confectioners' sugar
 1 cup sifted unsweetened cocoa
 ½ cup soy milk

Stir the sugar and the cocoa together in a bowl. Stir in the soy milk, mixing until smooth. Use immediately to drizzle over cooled cakes or cookies.

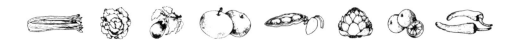

INDEX

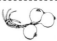

CLAIRE CRISCUOLO graduated from the University of Bridgeport in 1975 and is a registered nurse. Her love of good food, along with her desire to create exciting, home-cooked meals led her into the restaurant business only months after graduation. Armed with the recipes she culled from a family of marvelous cooks (Claire's mom continues to cook at her daughter's restaurant), she and her husband, Frank, founded **Claire's Corner Copia** in September, 1975.

Claire's Corner Copia is a vegetarian restaurant which continues to thrive at its original location across from Yale University and the historic Green in New Haven, Connecticut. Over the years, **Claire's Corner Copia** has received glowing reviews in local and national publications, including *The New York Times*, and has won top awards in the Best of New Haven contest held annually by the *New Haven Advocate*.

Dedication to quality has long been the mission at **Claire's Corner Copia**. The restaurant's superb reputation and tremendous success has provided it with the resources to give something back to the community. Every year **Claire's** collects thousands of dollars and donates it to a myriad of worthwhile causes. Among them are various AIDS projects, Easter Seals, Rachel's Table, Share Our Strength, battered women's shelters, soup kitchens, and other groups. Claire is a recipient of the Cy Flanders Award for her work with people with disabilities and the 1993 award from AIDS Project New Haven for outstanding community involvement.